T0358912

Gender and Diversity in Oral and Maxillofacial Surgery

Editors

FRANCI STAVROPOULOS
JENNIFER E. WOERNER

ORAL AND MAXILLOFACIAL SURGERY CLINICS OF NORTH AMERICA

www.oralmaxsurgery.theclinics.com

Consulting Editor
RUI P. FERNANDES

November 2021 • Volume 33 • Number 4

ELSEVIER

1600 John F. Kennedy Boulevard • Suite 1800 • Philadelphia, Pennsylvania, 19103-2899

http://www.oralmaxsurgery.theclinics.com

ORAL AND MAXILLOFACIAL SURGERY CLINICS OF NORTH AMERICA Volume 33, Number 4
November 2021 ISSN 1042-3699, ISBN-13: 978-0-323-81375-4

Editor: John Vassallo; j.vassallo@elsevier.com
Developmental Editor: Jessica Nicole B. Cañaberal

Oral and Maxillofacial Surgery Clinics of North America (ISSN 1042-3699) is published quarterly by Elsevier Inc., 360 Park Avenue South, New York, NY 10010-1710. Months of issue are February, May, August, and November. Business and Editorial Offices: 1600 John F. Kennedy Blvd., Suite 1800, Philadelphia, PA 19103-2899. Periodicals postage paid at New York, NY and additional mailing offices. Subscription prices are $401.00 per year for US individuals, $933.00 per year for US institutions, $100.00 per year for US students/residents, $474.00 per year for Canadian individuals, $984.00 per year for Canadian institutions, $100.00 per year for Canadian students/residents, $525.00 per year for international individuals, $984.00 per year for international institutions and $235.00 per year for international students/residents. To receive student/resident rate, orders must be accompanied by name or affiliated institution, date of term, and the *signature* of program/residency coordinator on institution letterhead. Orders will be billed at individual rate until proof of status is received. Foreign air speed delivery is included in all *Clinics* subscription prices. All prices are subject to change without notice. **POSTMASTER:** Send address changes to *Oral and Maxillofacial Surgery Clinics of North America,* Elsevier Periodicals **Customer Service, 11830 Westline Industrial Drive, St. Louis, MO 63146. Tel: 1-800-654-2452 (U.S. and Canada); 314-447-8871 (outside U.S. and Canada). Fax: 314-447-8029. E-mail: journalscustomerservice-usa@elsevier.com (for print support); journalsonlinesupport-usa@elsevier.com (for online support)**.

Reprints. For copies of 100 or more, of articles in this publication, please contact the Commercial Reprints Department, Elsevier Inc., 360 Park Avenue South, New York, NY 10010-1710. Tel.: 212-633-3874; Fax: 212-633-3820; Email: reprints@elsevier.com.

Oral and Maxillofacial Surgery Clinics of North America is covered in *MEDLINE/PubMed* (*Index Medicus*), *Science Citation Index Expanded (SciSearch®)*, *Journal Citation Reports/Science Edition*, and *Current Contents®/Clinical Medicine*.

Contributors

CONSULTING EDITOR

RUI P. FERNANDES, MD, DMD, FACS, FRCS(Ed)
Clinical Professor and Chief, Division of Head and Neck Surgery, Program Director, Head and Neck Oncologic Surgery and Microvascular Reconstruction Fellowship, Departments of Oral and Maxillofacial Surgery, Neurosurgery, and Orthopaedic Surgery & Rehabilitation, University of Florida Health Science Center, University of Florida College of Medicine, Jacksonville, Florida

EDITORS

FRANCI STAVROPOULOS, DDS
Associate Professor, Director, Undergraduate OMS Program, Department of Oral and Maxillofacial Surgery, Oregon Health & Science University, School of Dentistry, Portland, Oregon

JENNIFER E. WOERNER, DMD, MD, FACS
Associate Professor, Associate Dean of Academic Affairs, Tilakram and Bhagwanti Devi Distinguished Professorship in Cleft Lip & Palate Surgery and Training, Fellowship Director of Craniofacial and Cleft Surgery, Department of Oral and Maxillofacial Surgery, Louisiana State University Health Sciences Center Shreveport, Shreveport, Louisiana

AUTHORS

SHELLY ABRAMOWICZ, DMD, MPH, FACS
Section Head, Oral and Maxillofacial Surgery, Children's Healthcare of Atlanta, Associate Professor in Surgery and Pediatrics, Division of Oral and Maxillofacial Surgery, Department of Surgery, Emory University School of Medicine, Atlanta, Georgia

SARA HINDS ANDERSON, MS, DDS, MD
Department of Oral and Maxillofacial Surgery, Michigan Medicine, Ann Arbor, Michigan

RACHEL BISHOP, DDS, MD
Clinical Cleft and Craniofacial Fellow, Department of Oral and Maxillofacial Surgery, Louisiana State University Health Sciences Center Shreveport, Shreveport, Louisiana

LAUREN BOURELL, DDS, MD
Western Lake Erie OMS, Sylvania, Ohio

ANDREA B. BURKE, DMD, MD
Assistant Professor, Department of Oral and Maxillofacial Surgery, University of Washington School of Dentistry, Seattle, Washington

BRETT L. FERGUSON, DDS, FACS, FACD, FICD
Chairman, Department of Oral and Maxillofacial Surgery, University of Missouri–Kansas City, Associate Professor, UMKC

School of Medicine, Truman Medical Center, University Health, Kansas City, Missouri

LESLIE R. HALPERN, DDS, MD, PhD, FACS, FICD
Professor, Section Head, Oral and Maxillofacial Surgery, University of Utah, School of Dentistry, Salt Lake City, Utah

CATHERINE HAVILAND, DDS
Resident, Oral and Maxillofacial Surgery, University of Michigan, Ann Arbor, Michigan

PAMELA J. HUGHES, DDS
Associate Professor, Department of Oral and Maxillofacial Surgery, Oregon Health & Science University, Portland, Oregon

JUSTINE SHERYLYN MOE, MD, DDS
Clinical Assistant Professor, Residency Program Director, Oral and Maxillofacial Surgery, University of Michigan, Michigan Medicine, Ann Arbor, Michigan

MARIA MORGAN, JD
Chief Equity, Diversity and Inclusion Officer, Truman Medical Centers/University Health, Juris Doctorate, University of Missouri–Kansas City, Kansas City, Missouri

JANE A. PETRO, MD, FACS, FAACS
Professor of Surgery, Emerita New York Medical College, Valhalla, New York

FRANCI STAVROPOULOS, DDS
Associate Professor, Director, Undergraduate OMS Program, Department of Oral and Maxillofacial Surgery, Oregon Health & Science University, School of Dentistry, Portland, Oregon

SUSAN B. WILSON, PhD, MBA
Department of Diversity and Inclusion, University of Missouri–Kansas City, School of Dentistry, Kansas City, Missouri

JENNIFER E. WOERNER, DMD, MD, FACS
Associate Professor, Associate Dean of Academic Affairs, Tilakram and Bhagwanti Devi Distinguished Professorship in Cleft Lip & Palate Surgery and Training, Fellowship Director of Craniofacial and Cleft Surgery, Department of Oral and Maxillofacial Surgery, Louisiana State University Health Sciences Center Shreveport, Shreveport, Louisiana

Contents

> Oral and maxillofacial surgeons experience high levels of stress and work–home conflict, which predispose them to burnout. There is emerging evidence in support of work–life integration to prevent burnout; interventional strategies exist on an individual and organizational level. This article explores the current evidence on promoting work–life integration for improved surgeon satisfaction, performance, and efficiency. Work–life integration initiatives can help promote the recruitment and retention of a diverse surgical workforce in oral and maxillofacial surgery.

> The COVID-19 pandemic altered all facets of society on a fundamental level, impacting work, mental health, and family life. Female surgeons experienced gender inequity and bias before COVID; therefore, women in oral and maxillofacial surgery (OMS) were affected disproportionately by the repercussions of the pandemic. Well-established inequalities are intensified during times of crisis. This article enlightens readers regarding the preexisting inequalities in the OMS specialty, how the COVID-19 pandemic exacerbated these ubiquitous issues, and how the specialty should accommodate these inequities moving forward.

> Women emerged against significant obstacles in the nineteenth century to claim a right to participate in the health professions. Women were excluded from many areas of medical and dental practice until well after the 1964 Civil Rights Act forbade discrimination on the basis of sex. Their entry has been, and continues to be, blocked by discrimination, misogyny, and harassment both personal and institutional. The formation of women-specific surgical subspecialty organizations has improved access to mentoring, sponsorship, and acceptance. This article reviews the history of some of the older organizations with recommendations for OMFS women's action.

> Medical training in the United States has undergone multiple evolutions and maturations. The Flexner Report and its effects, written in 1910, still has significant impact on modern professional education in the medical and dental arenas. The National Academy of Medicine (Institute of Medicine) in 2003 documented the need for diversity in the health care work force, and the Association of American Medical Colleges likewise looked at Medical Education and endorsed workforce diversity. This article reviews diversification in the surgical trainee workforce.

The diversity bonus theorem developed by Scott Page postulates that in specific environments, diversity is an absolute necessity to creating the most successful team. The theorem dispels the myth that institutions must choose between diversity and excellence. Within oral and maxillofacial surgery, this bonus is captured through expanded access to care, more equitable and relevant research, and attracting the best and brightest to the specialty. To capture the bonus, oral and maxillofacial surgery must invest in policy changes to admissions and hiring practices, and offer training in communication, cultural competency, and implicit bias.

ORAL AND MAXILLOFACIAL SURGERY CLINICS OF NORTH AMERICA

SERIES OF RELATED INTEREST

Atlas of the Oral and Maxillofacial Surgery Clinics
www.oralmaxsurgeryatlas.theclinics.com

Dental Clinics
www.dental.theclinics.com

THE CLINICS ARE NOW AVAILABLE ONLINE!
Access your subscription at:
www.theclinics.com

Preface
Gender and Diversity in Oral and Maxillofacial Surgery

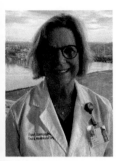
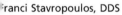
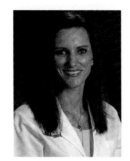

Franci Stavropoulos, DDS   Jennifer E. Woerner, DMD, MD, FACS

Editors

Oral and maxillofacial surgery emerged as a specialty in the first decade of the twentieth century and, sparked by scientific and technological developments, while being buffeted by social, economic, and political forces, has followed a winding path to its current robust status. Despite the specialty's many successes, diversity concerns have remained a perennial challenge. Ingrained traditions within professional education continue to inhibit progress toward equality among ethnic groups, women, LGBTQ, and people with disabilities. In this issue, authors explore the many dimensions of the problem and offer suggestions to aid in improving gender and diversity inclusion within the specialty.

We wish to thank Mr John Vassallo, Associate Publisher, Clinics Global Education, Elsevier, who recognized the need for examining and discussing gender and diversity concerns within the specialty. In addition, the editors and authors are indebted to Ms Jessica Cañaberal, Continuity Development Editor, Elsevier for her skillful assistance in the preparation of this issue. Most importantly, we are profoundly grateful to the outstanding group of authors who submitted relevant and consequential articles addressing gender and diversity concerns as well as methods to quicken progress toward betterment of the profession.

We dedicate this issue to Lucy Hobbs Taylor, the first woman in the world to receive a doctorate in dentistry. Despite rejections and setbacks, she completed her doctorate in dentistry in 1866 and practiced dentistry until her death in 1910. Her determination continues to be inspirational to us in challenging the gender and minority inequities in oral and maxillofacial surgery.

Franci Stavropoulos, DDS
Department of Oral & Maxillofacial Surgery
Oregon Health and Science University
2646 SW Upper Drive Place
Portland, OR 97201, USA

Jennifer E. Woerner, DMD, MD, FACS
Department of Oral and Maxillofacial Surgery
Louisiana State University
Health Sciences Center–Shreveport
119 Napoleon Drive
Shreveport, LA 71115, USA

E-mail addresses:
Mfstavro@gmail.com (F. Stavropoulos)
jennifer.woerner@lsuhs.edu (J.E. Woerner)

Oral Maxillofacial Surg Clin N Am 33 (2021) ix
https://doi.org/10.1016/j.coms.2021.08.006

Gender Issues and Oral and Maxillofacial Surgery Advanced Education Program Accreditation

Pamela J. Hughes, DDS

KEYWORDS

- Gender discrimination • Accreditation • Oral and maxillofacial surgery • Residency programs

KEY POINTS

- Women experience gender discrimination in the admissions process and during training in oral and maxillofacial surgery.
- Accreditation Standards for Advanced Education Programs in Oral and Maxillofacial Surgery do not address gender discrimination.
- Clear standards and processes need to be developed to ensure equity in our educational programs and to protect women from discrimination, harassment, and sexual violence.

It is undeniable that women oral and maxillofacial surgeons continue to encounter gender discrimination throughout their careers, and one of our most vulnerable groups to experience discrimination are the female oral and maxillofacial surgery (OMS) applicant and resident populations. In 2018, Rachel Uppgaard bravely shared some of her experiences as an OMS resident and as an OMS attending faculty member that were truly disturbing, yet unfortunately, not surprising.[1] One only needs to read the "examples of free text comments for ranking programs last or not at all" in the article by Lee and colleagues[2] to be outraged at the blatant disregard for general human decency, let alone employment law, by some of my colleagues during the resident application/interview process (**Box 1**). These instances are not the only examples of discrimination that women residents experience as they progress through their training in OMS. There are less obvious, implicit biases built into our systems that challenge women OMS residents. In a Journal of Oral and Maxillofacial Surgery editorial, Dr Laskin cited

family (child bearing/rearing) as a deterrent for women to enter the specialty of OMS.[3] It is no secret that the culture of OMS training historically has discouraged childbearing. Women residents are in prime childbearing age when progressing through their residency training; yet, programs never seem prepared to handle such a common, expected life event. Why should women be expected to put off having children and take on a high-risk pregnancy later so that it is more convenient for their residency program? Why do we expect women to delay family priorities until they are finished with residency? More importantly, why is it considered a burden and why do we continue to deny basic human nature? The answers to these questions are obviously multifaceted and rooted in a system built for the patriarchy that has not changed much over the years. The author recognizes that there are residency program directors who are working hard to ensure better equity in their programs, and that is admirable; however, this is not something that should be left to each program director to

Department of Oral and Maxillofacial Surgery, Oregon Health and Science University, 3181 Sam Jackson Park Road, Portland, OR 97239, USA
E-mail address: pamjhugoms@gmail.com
Twitter: @pamjhug (P.J.H.)

Oral Maxillofacial Surg Clin N Am 33 (2021) 429–433
https://doi.org/10.1016/j.coms.2021.05.003
1042-3699/21/© 2021 Elsevier Inc. All rights reserved.

Box 1
Examples of free text comments for ranking programs last or not at all (no identifiers were used)

Overheard irrelevant and hurtful comments about other residents and applicants.

They noticed that I am from a certain area of the country and assumed I would most likely stay in that area, then proceeded to say "What the "*" are you doing here?" in the middle of the formal interview.

During an externship, I was holding a light for a male chief resident in the ED and he told me to step in close, my chest was pushed up against his arm and he said in a sneering way "Wow getting fresh with me huh?" ...I applied and interviewed with the program because I knew that resident wouldn't be there anymore and I had really liked the program otherwise, but at the end of the day ranked the program last on my list.

Racist comments about my accent

In one program, the PD's first question to me was "your rank and NBME score are awful why should I take you?"

A group of first-year residents were attempting to be candid but ended up just openly denigrating their program. The candor was eye opening but also off putting

Old white male surgeon, in the presence of 3 or 4 other white male surgeons, asked at a round table interview how old I was, how he was surprised I wasn't married. "How would you manage having children during residency?" ...I wish I would have left the interview immediately or even asked for reimbursement for wasted airfare and hotel...

One program told all interviews and I quote "if you try and switch to a different specialty, I will go out of my way to 'f***' you." I ranked this program last.

I felt it was rude for an attending to spend a substantial amount of time pointing out his perceived flaws in a research study in which I had participated.

Every program was excellent and female friendly, I did not feel biased against, except one interviewer at one program asked me, "Why don't you just want to be a homemaker?" I did not rank them.

A resident from a program I had applied to asked why I hadn't come to extern at their program and then proceeded to tell me that they had call rooms externs stayed in that had great perks such as playboy magazines ...I could only laugh because I was the dental student in a group of residents. I declined the interview invite from that program.

A senior resident said if they had to do it over, they would go somewhere else.

The program director literally tapped his watch and said "I know how old you are. Tick tock, tick tock—you need to have kids sooner than later." ... It was incredibly uncomfortable, let alone illegal and reflected so poorly upon him and his program.

That said, every one of his interviewers acted similarly, so he wasn't alone in his poor behavior.

Asking me if I applied to MD programs only because I wanted an MD degree.

One faculty member asked me if I fell in love with a man and had a child with him. and he wanted to move to Saudi Arabia during residency, would I consider it? This was a hypothetical scenario and it was not asked of any other individual during the interview.

Program director made multiple comments regarding kosher diet in a demeaning fashion and had questions if I would be able to complete residency requirements due to religious practices.

When I was an extern, one resident asked me, while we were seeing an ED consult, if I wanted to 'go to the call room after and f***. I said no and he proceeded to ignore me for clinical duties.

Program director asking me if I would be willing to work on Saturdays despite my religious beliefs .... He was very wrong. I love my chosen specialty and I have never allowed my personal beliefs get in the way of patient care or make things difficult for my coresidents.

Was told women in the program weren't allowed to get pregnant during residency.

I did not even apply to certain programs in my favorite geographic location due to their malignant reputations.

I was on an interview where all other interviewees were male... A certain faculty member said he was going to be doing one-on-one interviews in his office, where he subsequently asked me strictly personal questions. None of the other applicants were asked personal questions by this faculty member, only why they wanted to be in the OMFS profession, what they wanted to eventually pursue. etc.

Telling me a particular program would like me because of my race.

The place was too much a party/boys club atmosphere and would not have fit my personality

As a dental class, we wrote reviews about each program we externed with and shared them with each other. One of my male classmates started a review saying that the program was

* definitely not for females, because they are misogynistic." I didn't bother applying to that program.

The strip clubs aren't really tasteful.

I was specifically asked by a female faculty member. 'Why do you feel you need to work if your spouse has a good career?* ...I did not rank their program.

Abbreviations: ED, emergency department; NBME, National Hoard of Medical Examiners; OMFS, oral-maxillofacial surgery; PD, program director.

From Lee JS, Ji YD, Kushner H, Kaban LB, Peacock ZS. Residency Interview Experiences in Oral and Maxillofacial Surgery Differ by Gender and Affect Residency Ranking. J Oral Maxillofac Surg. 2019 Nov;77(11):2179-2195; with permission.

navigate. There needs to be clear, consistent policies across all our programs that allow women to feel welcome, safe, and supported, and they should feel that they are allowed to thrive in the specialty of OMS, and these policies need to be enforced. It is acknowledged by the author that this language should include all minoritized individuals, and this is not the focus of this particular article.

To be funded by the US Centers for Medicare and Medicaid and for its graduates to be eligible for ABOMS certification, Oral and Maxillofacial Surgery Residency Programs require accreditation by the American Dental Association's Commission on Dental Accreditation. It seems logical that a reasonable place to start to address gender issues in OMS residency would be in our specialty accreditation standards. The author's review of the current accreditation standards for Advanced Education Programs in Oral and Maxillofacial Surgery does not necessarily find instances of discriminatory language or policies; but what is clear is that the bar is set pretty low for programs to comply when it comes to antidiscrimination. The Commission on Dental Accreditation (CODA) OMS standards[4] includes only a single sentence regarding antidiscriminatory language, and it is concerning resident selection in standard 5. This is not adequate. The author has been involved in many site visits both as a site visitor, and as a program director, ushering two programs through four accreditation site visits over a 15-year period, and never once has seen the aforementioned standard language challenged or even questioned. Ideally, programs should not have to be threatened with reporting requirements to implement and practice antidiscriminatory policies, but having guidelines

for programs to follow sends a message that our profession cares about this issue and that we are committed to encourage, empower, and protect women as they progress through OMS training and that their presence in our specialty is valued and not seen as a burden.

The notion that our accreditation standards are inadequate around this issue is an understatement; however, it is reasonable to question whether this is a failing of our academic system in general. Hupp cites two processes that impair impartiality in our accreditation system.[5] The first is the use of volunteer peers as site visitors in general, and the second is the way the site visitors gather information from residents as a peer or, in some instances, a friend of their program director, creating a climate of fear of retaliation.[5] The author acknowledges that there is a pathway for residents to make a complaint outside of the site visit; however, CODA is only beholden to investigate complaints that relate to the accreditation standards for the specialty.[6] As there literally are no standards related to gender discrimination or harassment, is CODA obligated to investigate or provide discipline to a program for such a complaint? Presumably, institutions are left to police this on their own; however, our standards do not even require that institutions have such policies in place or that the programs prove that they are upholding their institutional policies.

In addition, a potential conflict of interest exists in the creation of our standards. The AAOMS Committee on Education and Training (whose members are mostly academic OMS) traditionally has taken on the responsibility to review and craft standards that then are reviewed by the specialty's faculty section (whose voting members are program directors and chairs) before they are presented to AAOMS leadership and CODA for comments and adoption. The fact that most individuals that have a hand in the development of the standards also have an interest in their program's ability to achieve or maintain accreditation is a conflict. Furthermore, at the time of this publication, there was only one female member serving on the Committee for Education and Training and only one female AAOMS trustee. A lack of representation at all levels of our profession's leadership needs to be addressed to create a culture of inclusion and equity in our training programs and in our profession in general.

Let us explore the one standard that includes antidiscrimination language, standard 5. How does one show that the resident recruitment process was free of discrimination? Resident selection is one of the most difficult processes that a program director faces. All human beings have biases. Recognizing these biases or eliminating details that may trigger these biases are important to conducting fair resident selection. Creating a nondiscriminatory system that helps our program directors to do this is sorely needed. In addition, any person involved in the interview process (including current residents) should undergo implicit bias training and understand what is not acceptable behavior or questioning during the interview process. Those that do not think this is important do not belong in the interview and selection process, and those that exhibit sexist behavior in the process need to be held accountable. It should not have to be said that this idea of professionalism should not stop after interviews. Ideally, this should be a concept that is also embraced once the resident matriculates, continues throughout training until graduation, and beyond.

As our specialty seems so obsessed with the fact that women may reproduce while in training, let us consider the questions posed earlier in this article regarding pregnancy during training. Why is having a resident out on maternity leave seen as a burden? First, our programs are inherently small, and they tend not to be able to efficiently function without the presence of residents whether in clinic, in the operating room, on call, or performing administrative duties. Perhaps the reason they are small is that instead of a competency-based education, we have a temporal and requirement-based system that continues to assume that a certain number of procedures in different disciplines will ensure a resident is competent and that they will finish in the time prescribed. Requirement-based education makes it difficult for program directors to manage work-force issues when it comes to residents taking leave. For instance, if a resident takes extended leave for whatever reason, and needs to extend their training, that may put the program over their limit of accredited positions Currently, there is no standardized, predetermined pathway for that trainee to become an "additional" resident from an accreditation perspective. Each case is reviewed independently; a program may be cited for not having enough of a certain type of procedure given the additional trainee, and a reporting requirement or worse may be issued. If we are going to keep track of case numbers, perhaps a better use of such tracking would be to ensure gender case equity. A recent study published in the ophthalmology literature showed that male residents, on average, performed more cataract surgeries than their female counterparts, even if the female residents did not take any leave.[7] There does not appear to be any studies to evaluate this in our specialty; however, it should be required that

programs provide an equitable distribution of learning experiences for all matriculates. Second, our programs tend to be "at-risk programs" in the eyes of our Graduate Medical Education offices when it comes to duty hour restrictions. Our standards state that there must be OMS call coverage 24/7. The reality is that for many small programs, this is an unrealistic expectation given the aforementioned duty hours even when there is no resident taking leave. Nevertheless, when just one resident is on leave, a program may be at risk of violating duty hours, or worse, risk resident personal injury due to sleep deprivation. Not only is this burden difficult for the team members assuming the additional work, it is difficult for the person assuming the leave. The level of guilt to which the resident on leave assumes is unfair and unhealthy. Given that parental leave, in most instances, is not used equally (In the United States, fathers tend to not take as much leave.) sets up additional inequities not only during resident training but also in all areas of corporate or professional advancement.[8] Leave aside, when the resident returns from maternity leave, there also are no standards for facilities such as lactation space (or even allowing time for lactation), milk storage, and so forth. One may argue that the institution that sponsors the program must have these policies in place and that the accreditation process acknowledges that fact, but some do not. In addition, it is not routine that programs must prove that they are adhering to such policies. Minimal standards need to be set regardless of institutional guidelines.

Finally, the author wishes to address sexual violence, unwanted touching, stalking, bullying, or other forms of harassment. Keep in mind that institutions that receive federal funding are required to uphold Title IX. Hostile work environment is also covered under Title IX. "A work or learning environment is 'hostile' when unwelcome verbal, nonverbal, or physical behavior of a prohibited nature is severe or pervasive enough to unreasonably interfere with an employee's work or a student's learning, or creates an intimidating, hostile, or offensive environment. An employer, teacher, coworker, vendor, or fellow student can create a hostile environment."[9] If one again refers to the table included from the article by Lee and colleagues,[2] it is the authors opinion that a hostile environment is likely the most common form of harassment that women in our profession face. The accumulation of microaggressions has a significant effect on a resident's mental wellness and performance. This does not mean that physical forms of abuse or harassment are not happening. We must believe women, and we must do better when it comes to investigating claims of discrimination or harassment. We also need to empower and encourage our male residents to speak up and act as allies for their female counterparts. Strong standards need to be developed to ensure that women will be heard and that their claims will be investigated fairly and impartially. Again, it may be logical to think that sponsoring institutions should hold this responsibility; however, as seen again and again, cover-up and protection of the abuser has prevailed in many instances, and many of our institutions have failed women.

In closing, it is clear that our current OMS accreditation standards do not, for the most part, address gender inequity in OMS training and, in some instances, makes it challenging for our program directors who are committed to creating more inclusive, equitable programs. If our specialty truly is committed to diversity and inclusion, creating standards that reflect that commitment would be a good place to start.

DISCLOSURE

The author has nothing to disclose.

REFERENCES

1. Uppgaard R. Addressing Gender Discrimination in Oral and Maxillofacial Surgery via the Social Norms Approach. J Oral Maxillofac Surg 2018;76:1604–5.

2. Lee JS, Ji YD, Kushner H, et al. Residency interview experiences in oral and maxillofacial surgery differ by gender and affect residency ranking. J Oral Maxillofac Surg 2019. https://doi.org/10.1016/j.joms.2019.06.174.

3. Laskin DM. The Role of Women in Academic Oral and Maxillofacial Surgery. J Oral Maxillofac Surg 2015;73:579.

4. Accreditation Standards for Advanced Education Programs in Oral and Maxillofacial Surgery American Dental Association Commission on Dental Accreditation (ADA CODA). February, 2021.

5. Hupp J. Residency Program Accreditation—Possible Improvements. J Oral Maxillofac Surg 2020;78:177–8.

6. ADA CODA Evaluation and Operational Policies and Procedures. Available at: https://www.ada.org/~/media/CODA/Files/eopp.pdf?la=enManual.

7. Gong D, Winn BJ, Beal CJ, et al. Gender Differences in Case Volume Among Ophthalmology Residents. JAMA Ophthalmol 2019;137(9):1015–20. https://doi.org/10.1001/jamaophthalmol.2019.2427.

8. Zallis S. Men Should Take Parental Leave, Here's Why. Forbes. 2018. Available at: https://www.forbes.com/sites/shelleyzalis/2018/05/03/why-mandatory-parental-leave-is-good-for-business/?sh=4b3e91729ded.

9. Title IX: US Department of Education, Office for Civil Rights. Available at: https://www2.ed.gov/about/offices/list/ocr/docs/tix_dis.html.

The Odyssey of Mentoring "A Paradigm Shift from Baby Boomer to Millennial and Beyond"

Leslie R. Halpern, DDS, MD, PhD, FICD

KEYWORDS

- Mentorship • Gender and diversity • Mentorship models • Cultural competence • Implicit bias
- Mentorship in oral and maxillofacial surgery

KEY POINTS

- Within the last decade, the role of a mentor has undergone a metamorphosis from the traditional Halsteadian model to a more *"mosaic mentor"* with innovative strategies specific to the mentee's individual challenges.
- An effective mentor exhibits a degree of seniority, reputation, and experience to enhance the mentee's productivity for success; must be compatible on numerous levels with the alignment of values to ensure long-term success in their disciplines; and should not represent a position with possible conflicts of interests.
- A variety of mentoring models are beneficial within the surgical training environment due to time spent in the operating room, hours spent caring for patients, being on call, and innovations in technology, all of which the mentee must achieve for professional growth.
- There is a call to action, at the organizational level to provide formal training of mentors who will become adept in advancing gender equity, diversity, and cultural competence with not only their students, residents, and fellows but also the patient community that they serve.
- An approach using the "pipeline hypothesis "has the potential to increase enrollment and retention for women oral and maxillofacial surgeons to achieve academic success and professional growth.

INTRODUCTION

"We must acknowledge that the most important, indeed the only thing we have to offer our students is ourselves. Everything else they can read in a book" D. Tosteson, MD, Dean, Harvard Medical School[1] "(or find on the web"; L.R.H.)

The role of mentorship in surgery and its subspecialties has a long and well-celebrated heritage. Surgeons have an innate ability to appreciate, respect, and give "awe" to the contributions made by the icons in their field of expertise. The array of surgical texts regardless of specialty is abound with portraits, photographs, and famous pearls of wisdom from the trailblazers who forged a path for the legacies that followed. These leaders have either knowingly or unknowingly created the foundation of surgical mentorship and its rewards throughout the twentieth century and now twenty-first century. This author has been privileged as a "baby boomer" female to have gained knowledge from several quintessential mentors in the specialty of oral and maxillofacial surgery (OMFS).

My contemporary colleagues and I have continued to carry the "torch of mentorship" at the predoctoral, residency, and junior faculty developmental levels, and our community of mentee's have benefited didactically and clinically to attain the surgical knowledge for evidence-based patient care. A decade ago, Dr Leon Assael stated: "Mentoring is the single most powerful tool to the learning and practice of surgery."[2] Within the last

Oral and Maxillofacial Surgery, University of Utah, School of Dentistry, 530 South Wakara Way, Salt Lake City, UT 84108, USA

E-mail address: Leslie.halpern@hsc.utah.edu

Oral Maxillofacial Surg Clin N Am 33 (2021) 435–447
https://doi.org/10.1016/j.coms.2021.06.001
1042-3699/21/© 2021 Elsevier Inc. All rights reserved.

decade, the role of a mentor has undergone a metamorphosis from the traditional Halsteadian model to a more "mosaic mentor" with innovative strategies specific to the mentee. The contemporary mentor continues to be faced with the challenges of a new breed of oral and maxillofacial surgeons who are unique with respect to surgical skillsets, technology, gender, culture, lifestyle, and most importantly evidence-based standards for surgical success. Dr James Hupp in an OMFS editorial suggests "two-way mentoring" so that both parties are accountable with respect to their roles and responsibilities.[3] By doing so the mentee not only receives the positive impact from his or her mentor or mentors, but more importantly, attains the surgical knowledge to benefit the surgical care of their patients and future legacy of surgeons who will follow.

The definition of an odyssey can be both literal (a long wandering or voyage usually marked by many changes of fortune) and figurative (an intellectual or spiritual wandering or quest). This article will accompany the reader on an "odyssey" of surgical mentorship beginning with historic origins, followed by a series of definitions of what a mentor is and is not, the dynamics of evolutionary change in style of mentoring, and evidence-based studies in the tools now applied to mentor our future oral and maxillofacial surgeons. The changing demographics of trainees will be highlighted to craft a paradigm for mentorship that is unique for the mentee. Future directions for strategies of mentoring will be presented to effectively update the roles of the mentor and mentee in the specialty of OMFS.

LITERATURE SEARCH

A literature search was undertaken using Medline within the PubMed portal to choose articles within the last 30 years. Only articles in English were chosen for inclusion. The keywords chosen include "mentor," "surgical education," "surgery mentor," "mentorship," "history of mentorship," "oral surgery and mentoring," "mentorship in medicine," "mentorship in dentistry," and "role models and coaching." Further articles were extracted from commentaries across the subspecialties of surgery.

History/Evolution of Mentoring

The term "mentoring" has its origin within the Greek language and translates to "enduring."[1] The concept of mentoring dates back to 2600 BC during the reign of a Sumerian king named Gilamesh whose arrogance and benevolence lead to a superior form of leadership.[2] The word "mentor"

was written by Homer in "The Odyssey." Mentor was a friend and confidant of Odysseus and was given the task of teaching and guiding Odysseus' son Telemachus. Mentor's dedication to educate and watch over Telemachus provided an illustration of the concept of mentoring.[1,4] As Mentor became unable to advise well (or wisely/effectively), Athena assumed the role disguised as Mentor and played a significant influence on the ability of Telemachus to become an adult with the wisdom and capability of leadership.[1,4,5]

Surgeons of the nineteenth century provided a foundation for early surgical mentoring referred to as a "preceptorship" that was not really a framework for mentoring but was predicated upon the preceptor, one who was older and experienced.[1] Some treated their "preceptee's" as servants not quite ready to be independent, although trained. Theodor Bilroth was given credit as the true surgical mentor of this time. As the twentieth century followed William Halstead became the creator of a formal approach to surgical mentoring that forms the foundation we now follow. His interest in the emphasis on scientific evidence leading to clinical decisions is much of what today's surgeons follow as evidence-based practice in the clinical care of patients.[6]

In the 1950s and the 1960s with the rise of television there appeared numerous medical programs that depicted surgeons as "invincible mentors" to their younger disciples, that is, *Dr. Kildare* and *Ben Casey*. Shows like *Marcus Welby, M.D.,* gave the wide-eyed viewer (such as this author) a glossy career choice with only well-based intentions. Today's programming such as *Grey's Anatomy* project an alternative approach to mentorship and the demands that both mentors and mentee's face in their approach to patient care. The latter provides a stark contrast to the white male doctor depicted previously to a more contemporary role model (discussed later) with gender equality and physician educators across races and ethnicities. The demographics of surgical trainees in the twenty-first century is changing dramatically along with the diverse population being served (**Box 1**). With this in mind, there is now a shift in surgical mentoring with a framework for creative innovations and opportunities to enhance the personal and professional success of our mentees.[1,6]

Mentorship: Definitions and Distinctions

The medical literature, although abound with articles on mentorship, conveys that there is no one ideal definition of mentorship.[7–9] Healy and colleagues[6] in their review article of role models and

Box 1 Evolutionary changes in surgery		
	Twentieth Century	**Twenty-First Century**
Surgical demographics	Caucasian male	Gender diversity/ethnicity
Clinical schedule	Call every other night	80-h work week
Financial debt	Significant/payable	Payable over prolonged period
Patient care	Autonomous	Team based
Operative decisions	Unquestioned	Insurance based
Transparency/liability	Minimal accountability	Public information
Mentor	**Solitary**	**Multiple/fragmented**

Adapted from Rombeau J. What is Mentoring and Who is a Mentor? In: Rombeau J, Goldberg A, Loveland-Jones C. eds. Surgical Mentoring: Building Tomorrows Leaders. Springer Science + Business Media. Springer New York Dordrecht Heidelberg London, 2010: 1-14.

mentors in surgery use the definition of mentor provided by the Committee on Postgraduate Medical Dental Education in the United Kingdom as a "process whereby an experienced, highly regarded, empathetic person (the mentor) guides another (usually younger) individual (the mentee) in the development and reexamination of their own ideas, learning, and professional development."[9,10] The mentor should teach by example, encourage, motivate, promote independence, and rejoice in the success of their mentees.[11] Conversely, mentors must be cautious because their actions can be detrimental, that is, excluding the mentee from research publications, as well as threatening or refusing to write letters of support on their mentee's character and personal development. An example is rude behavior by a mentor to operating room staff in front of a resident that risks perpetuating that behavior by the resident. Negative mentoring, as such, has the potential to instill a significant lasting effect on a mentee that exceeds any positive mentoring that was experienced.[1,7,12,13]

EFFECTIVE MENTORS AND MENTEES
Mentor

The ideal mentor incorporates all the positive characteristics described previously. These roles, however, have become more complex and now encompass areas of work-life balance, personal development, and personal growth that is unique to each protégé.[14,15] Geraci and Thigpen[7] describe 3 parameters of an effective mentor: (1) one that exhibits a degree of seniority, reputation, and experience to enhance the mentee's productivity for success; (2) the mentor and mentee must be compatible on numerous levels with the "right chemistry" and alignment of values to ensure long-term success in their disciplines; and (3) the mentor should not represent a supervisory position with possible conflicts of interests.[16] The dynamics of effective mentoring include active listening, emotional support, and encouragement. Mentors must be prepared for lifelong learning, educational improvement, and professional growth along with their protégé. **Box 2** lists these parameters in greater detail.

Mentee

Historically, the mentee was known as a protégé (favorite), and the word was derived from the French verb protégér or to protect.[1] It is important

Box 2 Characteristics of effective mentors
1. Possess selflessness and commitments to mentee's success
2. Consistently demonstrates character, integrity, honesty, trustworthiness, ethics, and morality
3. Respects the mentee and mentoring relationship
4. Engages in self-reflection and demonstrates personal openness
5. Provides emotional support
6. Adept at active listening
7. Functions as a guide and facilitator rather than a director/dictator
8. Possesses knowledge of the institution, professional field, and academic culture
9. Is able to provide honest, constructive feedback in a supportive manner
10. Assists reflection
11. Keeps both parties accountable

Adapted from Geraci SA, Thigpen SC. A Review of Mentoring in Academic Medicine. Am J Med Sci. 2017 Feb;353(2):151-157; with permission.

to qualify the responsibilities of the mentee. The latter ensures the success and achievement of each's goals.[7,16,17] Mutual respect and communication between mentor and mentee are foremost. The mentee must be proactive from the outset to seek out a potential mentor or series of mentors. The selection is often based on expertise or academic standing, professional characteristics, and availability. The mentee is responsible for networking among peers and faculty as early as possible in one's professional career. This ensures that their productivity is noticed and appreciated by the potential mentor. This can also be referred to as *managing up*, that is, taking the "driver's seat" in the mentor-mentee relationship.[8,18] The mentee must make clear expectations and how the mentor will assess goals both in formative and summative metrics. Three key objectives are needed for success: (1) characterizing the anticipated goals of the mentorship, (2) characteristics of the participants, and (3) the structure of the mentorship program.[8] Ultimately, the mentees will find it advantageous to seek different mentors to address distinct aspects of their professional and personal life.

ROLE MODELS/COACHES/TEACHING

The following represent components of mentee support that when taken together comprise all the qualities of effective mentoring (**Box 3**):

Role Models

A role model is predicated upon the demonstration of "how to be a successful, high quality academic physician through example alone and may be passive on the part of the senior academician"[6–8,19,20]; it encompasses educators whose professional behaviors are mirrored by the mentee's aspirations of qualities they would like to have, as well as positions that they would like to reach. The surgical role model has evolved from a traditional demanding individual to a team leader with a strong reputation, professional authority, and substantial communication skills.[6,21] Studies have found that student's choice of surgery as a specialty is based on the presence of positive surgical role models. Residents exposed to these positive attributes maintain how the impact of words, actions, and attitudes become a part of their behavior, which perpetuates itself in the resident's responsibility to be a positive role model for their junior colleagues.[7,8,21] Although most mentors are role models, most role models are not mentors. The differences are related to the extent of the interaction (see later discussion).[1]

Coaching

Coaching is applied to impart a specific level of knowledge or to aid in the attainment of a defined goal. Coaching is directed by a task master (coach) who concentrates on this goal.[6,7,19] The qualities of coaching include aspects of mentoring, as well as teaching, and can form an intricate part in the training of surgeons because coaching focuses on improving and refining existing skills.[19] In surgical residency this approach is often done as a debriefing after the operative case, which involves facilitated reflection, feedback, defining

---

Box 3
Characteristics of effective mentors, teachers, and coaches

Mentors	Teachers	Coaches
Knowledgeable	Knowledgeable	Knowledgeable
Sincere	Expert communication skills	Strong interpersonal skills
Available	Approachable	Cultivate mutual trust
Stimulate enthusiasm	Passion for their subject area	Facilitate learner-directed development
Trustworthy	Good technical skills	Highly respected
Flexible	Adapted to different learning styles	Adapt approach to individual learner goals
Good listening skills	Good listening skills	Active listener
Challenge the mentee	Set clear objectives	Recognize the learner's abilities and experience
Evaluate their own effectiveness	Strong rapport with learners	Nonjudgment
Track record with other mentees	Organized	

Adapted from Lin J, Reddy RM. Teaching, Mentorship, and Coaching in Surgical Education. Thorac Surg Clin. 2019 Aug;29(3):311-320; with permission.

deficiencies, and emphasizing positive perfor-mance. Often technology is provided as an adjunct or technical skill assessment and feedback. The structural approach of coaching can be individual-ized to each trainee's needs and goals based on their level of training.[19,22–24] A coach has the po-tential to help the surgeon change his or her un-conscious deficiencies to conscious ones, as well as have a greater awareness of conscious abilities, thereby maximizing a mentee's potential.

Teaching

The evolution of teaching in both medicine and surgery has included innovative approaches that require independent study, research projects, and longitudinal patient experiences for the surgi-cal resident of the twenty-first century. The teacher-resident relationship in surgical training encompasses both a didactic and technical skill component. Teachers can now approach learning in a wide variety of venues and allow their students to be self-directed in what must be learned. Liter-ature in thoracic surgical resident education dis-cusses curricula that "Educates the Educator" and contains didactic text, video training, and learning management courses that both train the trainer and resident.[19,25]

MENTORING MODELS

Several models of mentorship have been imple-mented by health care institutions to train both their residents and faculty. **Box 4** lists the types and methods of delivery. Each model is predicated upon a need for different mentors for different ac-ademic goals, as well as personal develop-ment.[7,25–27] Although these models are beneficial within the medical community, the surgical training environment necessitates a unique approach. Reasons include time spent in the operating room, hours spent caring for patients, being on call, and innovations in technology to make surgi-cal intervention more cost effective and require more than a single mentor's experience. A study by Kibbe and colleagues[28] evaluated the number of mentorship programs in Surgery across the United States. Only half of the training programs actually had a formal mentorship program, and those that were formal did not have a structured approach, that is, lack of a structured curriculum, lack of formal training of the mentor, and appeal to only extroverted mentee's and limited commu-nication with others who would benefit from mentorship. The investigators concluded that given the importance of mentorship to career satisfaction and retention, development of formal mentorship programs should be considered for all academic departments of surgery.[28] A system-atic review by Entezami and colleagues[29] evalu-ated mentorship in surgical training by characterizing common themes of effective men-toring, as well as the barriers encountered. Bar-riers to effective mentorship included temporal difficulties, scarcity of qualified mentors due to a lack of mentorship training, and most significantly, a shortage of gender-matched mentors (see later discussion).[29,30] The investigators concluded that although mentoring of surgical residents has evolved since the Halsteadian/Socratic model, a formal mentorship program needs to be able to overcome the barriers mentioned. New ap-proaches include the ability to accept the ment-ee's individuality to motivate progress and advancement so that the success of the mentee builds on the success of the mentor. Future research should define the traits of a mentee that are desirable to overcome generational and cul-tural differences. Mentorship is a valuable art that must constantly be reassessed. The latter will pro-vide the strong empirical foundation for training quality surgeons.[29,30]

Mentorship and Gender

Contemporary studies on mentorship have called for an urgent need in advancing sex and gender equity across all surgical subspecialties. The persistence of gender inequity has perpetuated hindrance of female advancement, research op-portunities, and clinical practice.[31] Recent data in the United States and United Kingdom show that although the number of women entering the field of surgery is increased, many drop out due to life-style preferences. Yet other research has argued that the barriers of organization based on un-friendly work environments, gender discrimination, and "glass ceilings" prevent women surgeons ris-ing beyond a certain level of the surgical hierar-chy.[17,31,32] Female dental and medical students, as well as residents, agree that a mentor can have a significant impact on their career selection and advancement. For women identifying surgical role models, however, there exists a paucity of se-nior female mentors.[6,17,31,32] Such underrepresen-tation can consequentially impact both the practitioner and their patient pool, that is, research showed gender preference by female patients when compared with age-matched male co-horts.[33] Data from orthopedic surgical residency programs support sex-specific role models as prioritized much more often by women than by men (59% vs 29%; $P < .001$).[17,34] The investiga-tors state, however, that with so few women in or-thopedics and leadership positions, same sex

Box 4
List of models for mentoring and their approach

Mentoring Model	Type of Approach
1. Dyadic	The traditional mentoring model in which there is a one-to-one relationship; most common model that has influenced the progress of mentorship
2. Multiple	Similar to dyadic but the mentee is mentored by several mentors simultaneously and each mentor is facilitating the development of a particular area
3. Peer	Very collaborative and mutually beneficial, as the relationship is based on mentors, peers, or colleagues. The mentee may be able to share difficulties and questions to others at an equal level of knowledge as opposed to senior faculty
4. Distance-Web-based	For those at small centers who need expertise not available in home institution
5. Mosaic	Uses multiple mentors with different types of expertise concurrently or sequentially to satisfy the changing needs of the mentee
6. Functional	Help to complete a specific project or reach a well-defined goal; the mentor is chosen based on her or his specific goals and support interactions with academic promotion and other goals of mentee
7. Telementoring	Defined by use of communication technology to connect mentor and mentee by distance, that is, mentoring in the operating room by remote monitors to guide mentee's actions/skills

mentoring options are limited.[17,34] Several solutions to these dilemmas include active recruitment of diverse teachers, developing their skills as mentors, and providing mentoring strategies that incorporate cultural sensitivity to combat unconscious sex and ethnicity bias beginning in a pipeline fashion.[35,36] The latter affords an opportunity to encourage early interest among women and minorities, as well as provide continuous mentoring relationships whose foundation began during the early stages of predoctoral and resident education. Studies have focused on the gender gap with respect to the nonwhite woman surgeons and the lack of diversity of mentorship.[37] Frohman and colleagues[37] distributed a nationwide survey focusing on perception of salary, race, and discrimination in surgery and a lack of nonwhite women surgeons. Although there was only a 22% response rate, all the nonwhite women were satisfied with their career choice to become a surgeon; 20% of the respondents were persuaded by a mentor to enter the field of surgery, and the majority stated that the most negative influence on their decision was a lack of mentorship. Their results, however, substantiate that there is a lack of mentors to support the challenges of race, sex, salary wage gap in women, and ability to balance work and family commitments. The survey did show that nonwhite male surgeons earned the same salaries as their white male cohorts. A larger sample size is needed to address the inequities of a discriminatory work environment and salary gaps across gender and whether formal mentorship programs can help navigate through these inequities. Further recruitment strategies are proposed so that the number of female surgery mentors reflects the number of women pursuing surgical careers.[37] A systematic review by Hirayama and Fernando[33] identified organizational barriers to career progression of female surgeons with suggestions to facilitate career and job satisfaction. Organizational culture is a key barrier that forms the "glass ceiling" to hinder the progression of a woman's career.[33] The 2 factors most significant to female surgeon success were organizational culture and work-family conflict. The investigators propose that health care organizations and policy makers must support organizational facilitators that provide flexible pathways, more family-friendly working conditions, and most importantly role models and mentors in surgical specialties to change the culture of a male-dominated organization.[33,38,39] **Box 5** depicts the most common models of mentoring. Evidence-based data are still being measured and standardized across all specialties.[33,38,39]

Cultural Competency in Mentoring

As with sex and gender, health care providers are no longer a homogeneous cohort with respect to ethnicity and culture. Cultural diversity is a major issue due to the increase in international students, residents, and fellows in which intercultural communication is mandatory. As diversity is amplified in society, it is increasingly important for surgeons to be adept at interacting with patients from all backgrounds.[40,41] Mentors need to be especially adept at working with and understanding cultural differences/barriers with both their patient population and their mentees; this forms the basis of becoming culturally competent. Cultural competency is defined as "a set of congruent behaviors, attitudes, and policies that come together in a system, agency, or among professionals that

---

Box 5
Models of Mentoring for Gender

Dyadic mentoring model:

The dyadic model is the traditional and the most often successful mentoring model consisting of a one-to-one relationship. The dyadic approach is based on a male socialization (predominant in individual achievement), the sexual dynamics whereby a mentor of the opposite sex may or may not identify or understand a mentee's situation, opportunities and work style as a same sex mentor would. Women also tend to engage in equalizing behavior over hierarchical behavior. This model of mentoring, as such, may not be applicable to women as it is to men.

Multiple mentoring model:

This model is more applicable to female mentees by providing opportunities to establish a wider network in their field of expertise. An advantage of this model lies in having mentors who are in line with values and behaviors not only typical of females but also those associated with males.

Mosaic mentoring:

Mosaic mentoring uses multiple mentors with different types of expertise concurrently, or sequentially, to satisfy the changing needs of the mentee. A personalized mentor/advisor is chosen to identify and coordinate the mentee's relationships with clinical, research, and administrative mentors, of which some are themselves alumni of a mosaic framework.

Peer mentoring model:

This model provides collaborative approaches that are mutually beneficial among mentors, peers, and colleagues. A key aspect of this model is the lack of a hierarchal behavior/seniority, advantageous to some women due to their ability for equalization and willingness to collaborate for mutual learning, support, and expression of different perspectives. Innovative work styles can be crafted for flexibility between commitments to family and job responsibilities. Women can balance work-life challenges and advance their career aspirations

Data from Henry-Noel N, Bishop M, Gwede CK, Petkova E, Szumacher E. Mentorship in Medicine and Other Health Professions. J Cancer Educ. 2019 Aug;34(4):629-637.

enables effective work in cross-cultural situations…"[42]

Mentees who are cultural minorities face barriers because of the lack of identifying mentors with a similar cultural background.[42,43] Significant barriers include generational differences and a lack of instilled cultural competency. Both are synergistic because cultural differences are complex with respect to unique guidelines for approaching those "higher up," and if misunderstood, miscommunications can occur with unnecessary consequences. Frohman and colleagues[37] state "Trying to break stereotypes about having a foreign language accent in the Midwest male dominated program and lack of mentorship while feeling as an outsider." The latter if often a result of language barriers and so interpersonal communication is paramount to help the mentee to overcome his or her language barriers.

Cultural competence must begin at the institutional level, and all mentors need to be adept and open to diverse perspectives, values, and experiences.[44,45] A study by Aggarwal and colleagues[46] entitled "Is There Sex or Color Behind the Mask and Sterile Blue" examined sex and racial demographics across academic surgery by mining race and sex demographic data for all medical students, surgical residents, and faculty extracted from the American Association of Medical Colleges (AAMC) data files. Female surgery residents and faculty across all underrepresented ethnicities faced unequal barriers in pursuit of these goals. These barriers are likely rooted in years of "traditional" organizational culture that promote male domination and work-life pressure.[43,46,47] The lack of faculty mentorship from minority women further discouraged future women from seeing themselves in leadership roles. The investigators suggest some strategies that include building pipelines across universities to recruit minority students and increase the number of minority surgical faculty.[43,46,47] It is imperative that the administrators in positions of authority model positive behavior and promote inclusion.[46–49]

MENTORSHIP IN ORAL AND MAXILLOFACIAL SURGERY: WHERE ARE WE?

In 2010 a survey was sent to female practicing oral and maxillofacial surgeons, as well as residents, to define the changing personal and professional characteristics of women in OMFS.[50] The results showed that since 1994 there was an increase in the number of women entering the specialty. Barriers, however, included those discussed in previous sections, that is, sexual harassment and a feeling of exclusion; the field was still male dominant and imbalanced in

work/lifestyle matters and with "glass ceilings "to prevent academic advancement and leadership in educational settings.

In 2015, Dr Danial Laskin wrote a thought-provoking editorial in the Journal of Oral and Maxillofacial Surgery on the role of women in academic OMFS.[51] Although with good intention in stressing the importance of women as leaders and mentors, it failed to suggest solutions to foster a valid approach to enhance opportunities for women surgeons. There were several letters to the editor after D. Laskin's commentary that argued for a lack of understanding as to the true barriers of why there are gender gaps in work hours, male domination in positions of leadership, and lack of female mentorship. Dr Mary Delsol, former President of the American Board of Oral and Maxillofacial Surgery (ABOMS), stated this dilemma succinctly "...the ultimate goal is to recognize surgeons-not male, female, black, white or any other box…. The critical element is that there is equal opportunity…"[52]

An editorial by Dr James Hupp in 2015 provoked thoughtful arguments for how to train our future protégé's (mentees) on the merits of mentoring. OMFS is a highly desirable dental specialty only attracting applicants with a combination of intellect, work ethic, compassion, and dedication to serve others.[3] These qualities should be carefully groomed by the mentor to recruit future mentors. He goes on to describe the role of the mentor, which mirrors much of what is stated in previous sections of this article (see previous discussion). There is a call to action to enhance diversity and inclusivity of women and underrepresented minorities especially within the organizational framework of gender fluid mentorship and leadership in OMFS.[3]

A commentary by Uppgaard[53] in 2018 described a social norms approach to addressing gender discrimination based on personal experience.[54] This approach consists of recognizing misperceived attitudes by our colleagues and educating them to change their behaviors. When these perceptions are recognized then the observer/colleague will see them to be out of alignment with social norms and intervene to prevent future harm. The social norms approach has the potential to change the work environment and accept differences with a better understanding on the risk of damage from sexual harassment by colleagues. Zurayk and colleagues[55] created a study examining perceptions of sexual harassment in OMFS training and practice. The investigators concluded that sexual-based harassment was common in women oral and maxillofacial surgeons and recommend a curriculum to educate all esidents, faculty, and colleagues to ensure a safe environment for personal and academic growth. Faculty promotion and advancement in leadership at the organizational level continues to be a priority of the mentor-mentee relationship in OMFS. Mentor's should encourage women surgeons of all diverse backgrounds to seek teaching and leadership positions, integrate lifestyle, and establish long-term network relationships so that they may become mentors in the future and perpetuate a better work environment for their legacy. More importantly, mentors must support the need for diversity, inclusivity, and gender fluidity to close the gaps still present at the organizational levels of academic centers. Several questions are posed: (1) Why do women choose to enter academic OMFS?" (2)" Is gender associated with success in academic OMFS?" and (3) "Is there a need to develop pipeline programs to attract applicants from all gender and cultural backgrounds to provide a future of well-rounded mentors in OMFS?"

Kolokythas and Miloro[56] crafted question 1. An online survey consisting of 25 questions were sent via e-mail to all female oral and maxillofacial surgeons associated with an academic center. The responses were varied based on response rate, comfort in answering the questions asked as to reasons for women pursuing a career in academics, and what were the pitfalls for advancement. Of 84 e-mails sent, 31 completed the entire survey; 25 who were full-time and 6 who were part-time faculty. The investigators received a variety of reasons for choosing academic positions, that is, colleagues, collaboration, teaching residents, potential for research, and not being concerned with child rearing. Reasons for noninterest in academics include greater salary, being independent in decision making, more family time, and lack of institutional red tape. Most important were the lack of female role models and the importance of mentors who can recruit more females. Research should include ways to develop formal mentoring programs for female surgeons in academic centers and help to navigate the challenges faced by their younger female cohorts and provide possible solutions.

Burke and colleagues[57] crafted question 2. There exist disparities with respect to research and academic rank between female and male oral and maxillofacial surgeons that seem uniform across other surgical subspecialties. The premise was that academic success is predicated upon institutional rank, scholarship, and research opportunities. Their hypothesis and specific aims were to determine whether there exists a similar disparity between men and women with respect to academic rank and productivity as is seen in other surgical specialties. Their results were encouraging. There did not seem to be "gender bias" with respect to research productivity or academic rank among the full-time female OMFS faculty when compared with their male cohorts; this may have been due to the timelines of careers between the genders along with a continued mentorship pipeline for female dental students and faculty. Both are recognized for their exemplary achievements. The investigators do caution that future growth needs to be predicated upon shattering the "glass ceiling" with high-quality mentorship of women and a continued cognizant approach to diversity to change the culture of surgical mentees and reduce gender bias. The latter will forge a path for a greater presence of female and other underrepresented groups in OMFS.

The 2 questions mentioned earlier may be preceded by question 3. "Is there a need to develop pipeline programs to attract applicants from all gender and cultural backgrounds, as well as formal mentoring programs based upon diversity and gender"? A study by Lee and colleagues[58] examined data from dental school applicants in 2018 with respect to gender. More than 50% were female. In the same year of a pool of 1175 OMFS residents only 16.5% were female. Of the Fellows of AAOMS 8% were female and 92% were male. Although there has been an increase in the number of female oral and maxillofacial surgeons, they are still outpaced by females in other surgical subspecialties.[58,59] With the rise in female dental students more will consider OMFS as a career based on their interaction with residents and faculty mentors. Issues of a gender bias with respect to unprofessional behavior and race-specific questions not asked of male applicants prompted a study to evaluate the interview experience between females and their male cohorts to determine factors affecting the selection of programs and ranking based on the aforementioned assumptions. A total of 1134 surveys were sent to interviewees with a 14.6% response rate (165 respondents). The investigators concluded that although the sample was small, unprofessional behavior was more often experienced by female OMFS applicants, especially those applying to MD programs. The negative behaviors were from both residents and faculty interviewers with questions about pregnancy plans, relationships, and racial backgrounds. Such discriminatory behavior characterizes unprofessionalism that needs to be carefully monitored using the standards of the Commission on Dental Accreditation and the Accreditation Council for Graduate Medical Education (GMEC).

The implicit bias seen in the aforementioned study is a subtle enemy that needs to be eradicated by formal education of both residents and faculty. Numerous toolkits and courses are available through the American Dental Education Association (ADEA) and the AAMC. Lee and colleagues go on to suggest that diversity in committee members of different cultures and gender can level the field of selection of applicants for residency. Programs that are not diverse in faculty and residents may consider speaker selections for Grand Rounds that welcome females of all ethnicities and specialties to speak. This approach will build an interprofessional collaborative of gender and ethnicity that will change the culture at the organizational level. The latter should be composed of a mosaic of facilitators to coordinate the mentee's relationships with clinical, research, and administrative duties, personality conflicts, and work-life balance.

Barriers for advancement of gender equity in OMFS, as well as other surgical specialties, exist within a complex matrix of organizational and individual factors. Surgeon mentors within the specialty need to educate, elevate, and energize their residents and faculty to create a culture of

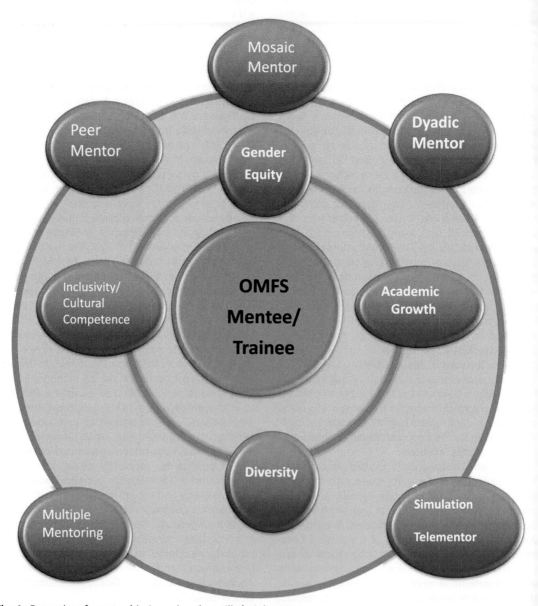

Fig. 1. Dynamics of mentorship in oral and maxillofacial surgery.

diversity and gender equity.[60] Dr MD Fahmy, oral and maxillofacial surgeon, states "Mentorship is indeed an essential element in oral and maxillofacial surgery education."[61] Formal programs should be brought to the table with operational resources to provide rewards for mentoring at the organizational level. This will provide "protected time" to develop mentorship strategies without anxiety of lost revenue, work-life balance, and productivity. Other models proposed include the development of "Pipeline "programs whose primary objective is to increase enrollment and retention of female OMFS faculty in the academic setting (A. Burke, personal communication, 2021). The benefits of mentorship will ultimately help to shape the future of OMFS by perpetuating a legacy of gender equity, diversity, strength, professional development, and growth (**Fig. 1**).

ACKNOWLEDGMENTS

The author thanks Dr Julianne Glowacki, Professor, Orthopedic Surgery, Oral & Maxillofacial Surgery, Emerita, Harvard Medical School and Harvard School of Dental Medicine, Scholar in Orthopedic Surgery, Brigham and Women's Hospital, Boston, MA, and Dr R. Wyatt Hume, DDS, PHD, Professor, Oral Biology and Dean of the University of Utah, School of Dentistry, Salt Lake City, Utah, for critically evaluating this article.

DISCLOSURE

The author does not have any relationship with a commercial company that has a direct financial interest in subject matter or materials discussed in the article or with a company making a competing product.

REFERENCES

1. Rombeau J what is mentoring and who is a mentor?. In: Rombeau J, Goldberg A, Loveland-jones C, editors. Surgical mentoring: building Tomorrows leaders. Springer Science + Business Media. Springer New York Dordrecht Heidelberg London; 2010. p. 1–14.
2. Assael L. Every surgeon needs mentors: A Halsteadian/Socratic model in the modern age. J Oral Maxillofac Surg 2010;68:1217–8.
3. Hupp JR. Two-way mentoring: Learning from residents. J Oral Maxillofac Surg 2020;78:1–2.
4. Sadoski SJ, Fitzpatrick B, Curtis DA. Evidence-based criteria for different treatment planning of implant restorations for the maxillary edentulous patient. J Prosthodont 2015;433–46.
5. The spiritual mentors of Boethius and Dante: the pagan spirit and the medieval love. Available at: https://johnledinghamprofessional.wordpress.com/2019/12/06/the-spiritual-mentors-of-boethius-and-dante-the-pagan-spirit-and-the-medieval-beloved/. Accessed November 26, 2020.
6. Healy NA, Cantillon P, Malone C, et al. Role models and mentors in surgery. Am J Surg 2012;204:256–61.
7. Geraci SA, Thigpen SC. A review of mentoring in academic medicine. Am J Med Sci 2017;353(2):151–7.
8. Henry-Noel N, Bishop M, Gwede CK, et al. Mentorship in medicine and other health professions. J Cancer Educ 2019;349:629–37.
9. Barondess JA. A brief history of mentoring. Trans Am Clin Climatol Assoc 1995;106:1–24.
10. Standing Committee for Postgraduate Medical and Dental Education. Supporting doctors and Dentists at work: an inquiry into mentoring. London: SCOPME; 1998.
11. Singletary SE. Mentoring surgeons for the 21st century. Ann Surg Oncol 2005;12:848–60.
12. Eby LT, Durley JR, Evans SC. Mentors' perceptions of negative mentoring experience: scale development and nomological validation. J Appl Psychol 2008;93:358–73.
13. Straus SE, Johnson MO, Marquez C, et al. Characteristics of successful and failed mentoring relationships: A qualitative study across two academic health centers. Acad Med 2013;88:82–9.
14. Atonoff MB, Varner ED, Yang SC, et al. Online learning in thoracic surgical training: Promising results of a multi-institutional pilot study. Ann Thorac Surg 2014;98(3):1057–63.
15. Sambunjak D, Marusic A. Mentoring: What's in a name? J Am Med Assoc 2009;302(23):2591–2.
16. Detsky AS, Baerlocher MD. Academic mentoring: how to give it and how to get it. J Am Med Assoc 2007;297(19):2134–6.
17. Mulcahey MK, Waterman BR, Hart R, et al. The role of mentoring in the development of successful orthopedic surgeons. J Am Acad Orthop Surg 2018;26(123):463–71.
18. Zerzan JT, Hess r, Schur E, et al. Making the most of a mentor: a guide for mentees. Acad Med 2009;84(1):140–4.
19. Lin j, Reddy RM. Teaching, mentorship, and coaching in surgical education. Thorac Surg Clin 2019;29:311–20.
20. Fagan M. The term mentor: A review of the literature and a pragmatic solution. Into J Nurse 1988;2:508.
21. Niihau's P. why should young doctors choose to become surgeons? Ann Surg 2007;246:911–5.
22. Bonrath EM, Dedy NJ, Gordon LE, et al. Comprehensive surgical coaching enhances surgical skill in the operating room: a randomized controlled trial. Ann Surg 2015;262(2):205–12.
23. Greenberg JA, Joiles S, Sullivan S, et al. A structured extended training program to facilitate

adoption of new techniques for practicing surgeons. Surg Endosc 2018;32(1):217–24.

24. Shubeck SP, Kanters AE, Sandhu G, et al. Dynamics within peer-to-peer surgical coaching relationships: early evidence from the Michigan Bariatric Surgical Collaborative. Surgery 2018;164(2):185–8.

25. Asuka ES, Halari CD, Halari MM. Mentoring in medicine: A retrospective review. ASRJETS 2016;19(1):42–52.

26. Owens BH, Herrick CA, Kelly JA. A pre-arranged mentorship program: Can it work long distance? J Prof Nurs 1998;14(2):75–84.

27. Wu JT, Wahab MT, Ikbal MF, et al. Toward an interprofessional mentoring program in palliative care-a review of undergraduate and postgraduate mentoring in surgery, medicine, nursing and social work. J Palliat Care Med 2016;6(6):1–14.

28. Kibbe MR, Pellegrini CA, Townsend CM Jr. characterization of mentorship programs in departments of surgery in the United States. J Am Med Assoc 2016;151(10):900–6.

29. Entezami P, Franzblau LE, Chung KC. Mentorship in surgical training: a systematic review. Handchirurgie 2012;7:30–6.

30. Muller MG, Karamichalis J, Chokshi N, et al. Mentoring the modern surgeon. Bull Am Coll Surg 2008;93(7):19–25.

31. Thompson-Burdine JA, Telem DA, Waijee JE, et al. Defining barriers and facilitators to advancement for women in academic surgery. JAMA Netw Open 2019;2(8):e1910228.

32. Desai A, Troulis MJ, August M. Evaluating the role of mentorship on women pursuing a career in oral and maxillofacial surgery. J Oral Maxillofac Surg 2020;78(10 Supplement):e.83–4.

33. Hirayama M, Fernando S. Organizational barriers to and facilitators for female surgeons' career progression: A systematic review. J R Soc Med 2018;111(9):324–34.

34. Hill JF, Yale A, Zurakowski D, et al. Resident's perceptions of sex diversity in orthopedic surgery. J Bone Joint Surg Am 2013;95:e1441–6.

35. Mason BS, Ross W, Ortega G, et al. Can a strategic pipeline initiative increase the number of women and underrepresented minorities in orthopedic surgery? Clin Orthoped Relat Res 2016;74:1979–85.

36. Van Heest AE, Agel J. The uneven distribution of women in orthopedic surgery resident training programs in the United States. J Bone Joint Surg Am 2012;94:e9.

37. Frohman HA, Thu-Hoai C, Nguyen BS, et al. The nonwhite woman surgeon: A rare species. J Surg Educat 2015;72(6):1266–71.

38. Jerg-Bretzke L, Limbrecht K. Where have they gone? - a discussion on the balancing act of female doctors between work and family. GMS Z Med Ausbild 2012;29:2.

39. Mayer AP, File J, Ko MG, et al. Academic advancement of women in medicine: do socialized gender differences have a role in mentoring? Mayo Clin Proc 2008;83(2):204–7.

40. Fiscella K, Frankel R. Overcoming cultural barriers: International medial graduates in the United States. J Am Med Assoc 2000;283:1751.

41. Koury A, Mendoza A, Charles A. Cultural competence: why surgeons should care. Available at: https://bulletin.facs.org/2012/03/cultural-competence-why-surgeons-should-care/. Accessed December 28, 2020.

42. Centers of disease control and prevention (CDC). Cultural competence in health and human services. Available at: https://npin.cdc.gov/pages/cultural-competence. Accessed October 21, 2020.

43. Patel SI, Rodriguez P, Gonzales RJ. The implementation of an innovative mentoring program designed to enhance diversity and provide a pathway for future careers in healthcare related fields. J Racial Ethn Health Disparities 2015;2:395–402.

44. Rombeau J, Goldberg A, Loveland-Jones C. Future directions. In: Rombeau J, Goldberg A, Loveland-jones C, editors. Surgical mentoring: building Tomorrows leaders. Springer New York Dordrecht Heidelberg London: Springer Science + Business Media; 2010. p. 145–64.

45. Welch J, Jimenez HL, Walthall J, et al. The women in emergency medicine mentoring program: An innovative approach to mentoring. J Grad Med Educat 2012;4(3):362–6.

46. Aggarwal A, Rosen CB, Nehemiah A, et al. Is there color or sex behind the mask and sterile blue? Examining sex and racial demographics within academic surgery. Ann Surg 2020;273:21–7.

47. Nellis JC, Eisele DW, Francis HW, et al. Impact of a mentored student clerkship on underrepresented minority diversity in otolaryngology–head and neck surgery. Laryngoscope 2016;126:2684–8.

48. Maina IW, Belton TD, Ginzberg S, et al. A decade of studying implicit racial/ethnic bias in healthcare providers using the implicit association test. Soc Sci Med 2018;199:219–29.

49. Available at: https://www.merriam-webster.com/dictionary/odyssey. Accessed December 25, 2020.

50. Rostami F, Ahmed A, Best AM, et al. The changing personal and professional characteristics of women in oral and maxillofacial surgery. J Oral Maxillofac Surg 2010;68:381–5.

51. Laskin D. The role of women in academic oral and maxillofacial surgery. J Oral Maxillofac Surg 2015;579.

52. Letters to the editor. J Oral Maxillofac Surg 2015. Available at: https://doi.org/10.1016/j.joms2015.03.075. Accessed December 24 2020.

3. Uppgaard R. Addressing gender discrimination in oral and maxillofacial surgery via the social norms approach. J Oral Maxillofac Surg 2018;76:1604–5.

4. Berkowitz AD. Fostering healthy norms to prevent violence and abuse: the social norms approach. In: Kaufman K, editor. The prevention of sexual Violence: a practitioners Source book. Holyoke, MA: NEARI Press; 2010. p. 147–72.

5. Zurayk LF, Cheng KL, Zemplenyi M, et al. Perceptions of sexual harassment in oral and maxillofacial surgery training and practice. J Oral Maxillofac Surg 2019;77:2377–85.

6. Kolojythas A, Miloro M. Why do women choose to enter academic oral and maxillofacial surgery? J Oral Maxillofac Surg 2016;74:881–8.

57. Burke A, Cheng KL, Ha JT, et al. Is gender associated with success in academic oral and maxillofacial surgery? J Oral Maxillofac Surg 2019;77:240–6.

58. Lee JS, Yisi DJ, Kushner H, et al. Residency interview experiences in oral and maxillofacial surgery differ by gender and affect residency ranking. J Oral Maxillofac Surg 2019;77:2179–95.

59. Available at: https://www.aamc.org/download/321442/data/factstableal.pdf. Accessed December 31, 2020.

60. Available at: http://htpps://bulletin.facs.org/2019/04/surgeon-leaders-need-toeducate-elevate-energize-to-create-a-cukture-of-diversity-an-interview-with-dr-julie-freischlag. Accessed December 27, 2020.

61. Fahmy MD. Mentorship: an essential element in oral and maxillofacial surgery education. J Oral Maxillofac Surg 2019;77:9–10.

The Gender Pay Gap in Oral Surgery

Lauren Bourell, DDS, MD

KEYWORDS

- Gender • Pay gap • Compensation • Inequality

KEY POINTS

- Gender inequality in compensation, the so-called pay gap, is pervasive across professions, including health care.
- Gender discrimination and implicit bias contribute to inequality in the workplace, both in pay and in advancement opportunities.
- Women are under-represented in many surgical specialties, including oral and maxillofacial surgery.
- Recognition of the gender pay gap is essential as part of a larger strategy to build equality and excellence in surgery.

INTRODUCTION

It seems self-evident that in the twenty-first century, compensation in the professions would be based on relevant skills and experience. It is expected that personal characteristics, such as educational background, influence salary but not personal attributes, such as gender, race, and religion. It may be surprising and disappointing, therefore, to admit that this is not the case. Women working in the same jobs as men make less money. This is true historically and up to the present day. It is true across wide-ranging disciplines, such as education, law, government, and health care. Women make less than men after controlling for years of experience, number of hours worked, job setting, medical or surgical specialty, and other factors.

This gender inequality extends beyond pay. Women also have fewer leadership roles and journal publications than do men. In academic medicine, women represent only 8% of surgery faculty.[1] In peer-reviewed journal publications, women authors are in the substantial minority.[2]

SCOPE OF THE PROBLEM
Historical Perspective

In the general workforce, women make approximately 82 cents on the dollar compared with men.[3] In medicine, the discrepancy is similar. Some of the earliest studies to examine this gender pay gap in health care were conducted in the 1970s. Two in particular reported a difference in earnings of 19%[4] to 24%[5] between men and women. A 1982 study[6] reported a difference in pay by gender of approximately 12% to 13%, which gave the impression that things were improving with time. A close reading of that study, however, reveals that the overall gender pay gap actually was 30%, but there was only 12% to 13% of that gap that the study investigators could not account for. That this "unexplained" gap was smaller than previous studies the investigators attribute to the improved mathematical functions they utilized to arrive at these numbers. The investigators concluded that some of the observed pay gap was based on differences in physician experience (ie, men had more years of experience) and higher-paying specialties (ie, more men in higher-paying specialties). The study investigators found, perhaps not surprisingly, that specialization and being board certified increased hourly earnings for both male physicians and female physicians. What is surprising, however, is that the increase was greater among women than men—women who were board certified in their specialty earned 25% more than nonboard certified women, whereas the earning advantage of board

Western Lake Erie OMS, 5690 Monroe Street, Sylvania, OH 43560, USA
E-mail address: lgb231@nyu.edu

Oral Maxillofacial Surg Clin N Am 33 (2021) 449–455
https://doi.org/10.1016/j.coms.2021.05.004
1042-3699/21/© 2021 Elsevier Inc. All rights reserved.

certification for men was 14%. The study investigators concluded with their expectation that over time the gender wage gap would decline, due to increases in female physician years of experience as well as increasing numbers of women going into higher-paying specialties. This has not occurred.

Current Data

Studies done as recently as 2016 and 2017 suggest that the gender pay gap in health care remains between 20% and 30%.[7,8] Many of these studies, particularly earlier studies, were based on surveys of self-reported physician income. More recent studies have made use of Medicare payment databases to provide a more objective quantification of the gender pay gap—these studies continue to affirm that the pay gap is real.[9]

Women have made great strides in the workplace since the 1970s and now are represented in fields and positions that previously were male-dominated. The proportion of women making up the entering classes of medical and dental schools has increased with each decade, such that there now is parity with men or occasionally even a female preponderance. This makes the persistence of a gender pay gap slightly more perplexing.

Perhaps most surprising is the finding that the pay gap actually gets bigger with time. A 2012 Yale University study[10] reports that women earn 13% less than men at the beginning of their careers. Eight years later, the difference grows to 28%. If, as some have suggested, the pay gap can be explained by a greater proportion of male physicians having more experience, it would be expected that the longer women are in the workforce the smaller the pay difference would become. The Yale study finds the opposite, suggesting that whatever factors account for the gender pay gap they operate independently of work experience. The fact that the pay gap is magnified over time suggests that not only are women paid less when first hired to a position but also they do not receive the same advancement, raises, and bonuses as their male counterparts. This reflects a problem not only with hiring practice but also with employee evaluation and advancement.

A 2015 study of physicians in academics found discrepancies in the number of women who were full professors compared with men—less than 50% of women compared with 61% of men. In academic surgery, the difference between women and men achieving full professorship is 18%.[11] This finding holds true in European countries as well, where fewer women attain permanent positions and positions of authority, such as senior consultant, department head, and section head.[12] In addition, men are promoted to these positions sooner than women and in higher proportion. Decades ago, when the overall numbers of women in medicine and surgery were small, it was easier to point to this as a reason for the small numbers in leadership positions. Now that the numbers of women entering and graduating from medical and dental schools is far greater, the absence of women advancing into the leadership hierarchy can only indicate that they remain at lower positions or leave academics entirely, the so-called leaky pipeline theory.

EXPLAINING THE GENDER PAY GAP
Conventional Wisdom

There are a variety of explanations for the gender pay gap which, although thoroughly debunked, continue to surface erratically in the popular press or physician news groups. These explanations for women's differential pay suggests that perhaps no pay gap exists or that if a gap exists it can be explained by factors that are concrete, reasonable, and not discriminatory. These include that women work fewer hours than men or that, if they work similar hours, they are less efficient and see fewer patients. There are suggestions that women may practice a more limited scope, manage patients more conservatively (ie, perform fewer procedures), or be less popular and less requested among patients. These possible explanations, although not implausible, have been carefully controlled for and ruled out as major factors in a large number of carefully designed research studies. Because people tend to personalize their experiences, it would not be surprising or necessarily wrong to count some of these as factors in the observed gender pay gap of a particular individual or group. It is more dangerous to apply this thinking with a broad stroke. Although a particular woman may work fewer hours than her male colleagues in the workforce overall, that cannot be the answer to the persistent gender pay gap, which cuts across nearly every profession in the United States and abroad.

Specialty Choice

Women are more prevalent in lower-paid medical specialties, such as general practice, pediatrics, and psychiatry.[13] Women also are rare in highly-paid specialties, such as orthopedic surgery and neurosurgery. Many of these lower-paying specialties are genuinely appealing to women, and no one would suggest that financial compensation is the only or even the main determinant in career path choice. It also may be true that female medical students are encouraged into specialties that require more of an empathetic, nurturing approach, such as psychiatry. It also can be easier for students to find a female mentor in a specialty, such as pediatrics, where women are well-represented. Mentorship increasingly is recognized as an important factor for students and trainees to realize their career goals. Women are not well-represented among the faculty and department chairs of surgical programs, and this may represent a barrier to female medical students choosing those specialties. If female students feel discouraged in pursuing a particular specialty, or if there is a lack of suitable mentors, they are unlikely to pursue that career path.[14]

Observational studies suggest that beginning in medical school, female students encounter gender discrimination from patients, staff, and supervisors.[15] These medical students report being ill-equipped to deal with gender bias, particularly from supervisors, and to becoming resigned over time to gender discrimination. This has been shown to affect these students' choices of medical specialty, particularly because fields with greater numbers of female patients or female supervisors are perceived to provide higher satisfaction.

Even women who choose surgery as a specialty are more prevalent in the lower-paid surgical specialties, such as obstetrics/gynecology and breast surgery (50%–60%). In traditionally male surgical specialties, the numbers are much lower—orthopedic surgery and neurosurgery (5%–8%)[13] and oral and maxillofacial surgery (5%–7%). Women are drawn to specialties like obstetrics and breast, where the patient population is female. It certainly is understandable that most women would prefer a female gynecologist or a female breast surgeon. This does not readily explain why women are not as highly represented in other surgical specialties. A study by Cochran and colleagues[16] surveyed surgical residents and junior faculty to ascertain what barriers to an academic career might exist. The biggest differences they found between the responses of men and women was that women were more likely to feel that gender discrimination and conflicts between having and raising children and their career were likely to have a negative impact on their advancement, whereas men did not.[16] The study also found that academic female surgeons are less likely to be married and less likely to have children than both their male counterparts and women in other medical specialties or other professions. Child-bearing status has been shown to have a negative correlation on income in at least 1 study.[17] Perceived in this way, it is not hard to imagine how female students might be reluctant to choose a specialty with a potential

for uncomfortable, discriminatory, or even hostile interpersonal interactions. When this type of workplace also includes significant challenges, real or perceived, to a satisfying family life, it can begin to be seen how surgery fails to attract women. What cannot be afforded to neglect, however, is that mutual respect and a collegial work environment are important to men and women both. The issue of work-life balance, particularly regarding children and families, often has been regarded as a women's issue. This is short-sighted—these are issues that affect everyone.

GENDER STEREOTYPES AND IMPLICIT BIAS

Although a small portion of the gender pay gap in medicine and surgery can be explained by clustering of women in lower-paying specialties, a more complete analysis requires considering the gender issues that operate more systemically. Blatant discrimination against women has not been tolerated for several years, thankfully, but gender bias continues to operate in the background of interactions in a much more covert fashion. This usually is not intentional but proceeds from a set of ideas about gender that are so normative that most do not recognize or critically consider them. A person's gender expectations are learned early in life as a part of cultural upbringing and become part of the mental background. This makes discrimination subtle, difficult to perceive, and challenging to change.

Men traditionally have been viewed as more task-oriented and authoritative. Their leadership style is more directive. Women are credited with being empathetic, nurturing, and collaborative. Women's leadership styles usually are less assertive and more team-oriented. Certain professions, including surgery, require characteristics that go against gender expectations. For women, an assertive leadership style often clashes with gender norms. Individuals may react strongly to an assertive woman, focusing on tone of voice, word choice, or perceived attitude as negative and undesirable. Some of these individuals are reacting to a woman who is behaving in a way that simply is unexpected. It creates a cognitive dissonance with underlying expectations. Without being aware of implicit gender bias, it is all too easy to label an assertive woman by a variety of uncomplimentary names.

Because discrimination against women is subtle and covert, it is tempting to believe it does not exist. Male surgeons and female surgeons both have a tendency to disavow that gender discrimination exists. One study involved focus groups and individual interviews of women in academic surgery.[18] The study found that although gender discrimination was pervasive, many women were openly dismissive of gender discrimination or tended to minimize the effect it had on their career advancement and satisfaction. To the study investigators, the situations these women described obviously were discriminatory, but it was clear to them that female surgeons did not want to be viewed as victims. There was a tendency for female surgeons to describe incidents of discrimination as being related to particular personal circumstances and, therefore, not as part of a pervasive system of covert and subtle bias.

In many professions, including surgery, there is a focus on success as being individualistic. The emphasis that personal qualities lead to achievement points away from systemic factors that may lead to success or failure. It tends to be believed that the hard work and perseverance of an individual lead to success, not social, cultural, or gender issues operating in the background of institutions. This individualistic focus is especially prominent in a field like surgery, which is highly competitive and where sustained academic achievement is necessary for success. Focus on the individual, however, makes it harder to identify the background issues, which are pervasive in the culture.

When it is recognized that the gender pay gap affects individuals at all stages of their careers across nearly every profession, it can begin to be understood that the causes and, therefore, the solutions also must operate at a systemic level. If success, both financial and otherwise, operated solely at the level of the individual, it would be expected the aggregate of individual outcomes to cancel each other out over time. Instead, what is found is a persistent trend in unequal pay for women. This requires that focus is shifted from the achievement of individual women and the system of renumeration and career advancement viewed through the lens of gender discrimination. Recognizing the patterns is the important first step toward creating a more equitable workplace.

GENDER DIFFERENCES IN EMPLOYMENT NEGOTIATION

Gender discrimination can negatively affect women's opportunities in the workplace, but women themselves not always are equipped to advocate for their own advancement. Dr Caprice Greenberg, in her 2017 Presidential Address for the Association for Academic Surgery, discussed differences in how men and women view success and how this has an impact on their career prospects.[19] Her remarks included ideas set forth in a book by Virginia Valian,[20] which explains that men generally attribute their success to their own ability. Men also consider that their failures are due to bad luck or great difficulty or a combination of factors. Women are more likely to relate their success to good luck or good timing. Women also may credit their failures to a lack of ability. This suggests that men more readily build confidence from their successes because they take full credit for them. Women may take less credit for their success and may carry more of the blame for their failures, resulting in more difficulty building confidence. Ironically, a recent study concluded that patients of female surgeons have better surgical outcomes than patients of male surgeons.[21] If women do have lower confidence than men, there certainly seems to be no reason for it.

Confidence is essential in many careers but certainly in the surgical specialties. It also is an asset when interviewing for a residency position, job opening, or a promotion. Confidence in skills as a surgeon also is an important factor in job satisfaction as well as the willingness to try new techniques or pioneer new procedures. If men and women build confidence differently, this suggests that an opportunity may exist in the mentorship and training of medical students and residents. At the very least, it suggests that the more objective standards can be implemented to measure success and failure, the better physicians can be equipped with concrete information to mediate extremes of either type, whether excess credit or excess blame.

One of the key areas where gendered constructions of success are especially impactful is in salary negotiation. Relative to men, women often place less emphasis on salary negotiations. There is a tendency for women to undervalue themselves and to ask for less money. Women also may place more emphasis on intangible items, such as work environment, support for research, or flexible hours. Women often are less effective at negotiating, and they can be judged more harshly if playing hardball about pay is viewed as aggressive. American culture frequently is uncomfortable with frank discussions of money and salary, and aggression is poorly tolerated from women.

GENDER EXPECTATIONS AMONG PATIENTS

Gender expectations operate at all levels of society, including academic institutions, hospital administrations, and individual patients. Patients generally are free to choose their doctors and some, or perhaps many, prefer male surgeons. It is a common scenario for a young female doctor to be told by a patient that they "look too young to be a doctor." In oral surgery, female surgeons may be asked if they are strong enough to extract teeth. There is much advice that has been given about tactful, humorous, or coy answers to these patient comments, but the fact that all these questions are oblique ways that patients have of asking about a female doctor's ability should not be overlooked. Youth and strength are observable traits that stand in for competence in a patient's mind. That women more than men should be fielding these questions speaks volumes about the social and cultural determinants of competence as well as the ways in which gender stereotypes have strongly affected the health care profession. In popular conception, as seen in movies, books, and TV shows, if not in real life, doctors often are portrayed as masculine authority figures. Female characters often are present in the secondary role of nurses. When female doctors are portrayed, they typically fulfill many of the feminine stereotypes of physical beauty and deference to male authority figures.

Many patients may seek these same masculine qualities in their doctors, without realizing that this is a gendered preference. The female doctor, although equally competent, likely is a less physically imposing presence. Patients may not recognize this expectation consciously, but it is revealed in questions about age or strength. Some patients may find physical size and strength to be comforting, especially if illness or debility makes them feel vulnerable. Some of the language used in health care, which describes fighting or battling against diseases, might suggest a need for strength. If patients do prefer a male doctor, then this is a potential explanation for the greater financial success of male physicians. This is unlikely to be the entire cause of the gender pay gap, but when it is considered that ancillary staff and administrative staff may share the same cultural biases as patients, it begins to be seen how subtle patterns of patient preference and staff bias could lead to scheduling differences, which, over time, could affect compensation.

GENDER AND FAMILY LIFE

Women may be reluctant to take on advancement opportunities at work due to perceived conflict with family duties. Women in most households perform the bulk of childcare and other household chores, and this is known to affect their attendance and advancement in the workplace. Disruptions in the availability of childcare have a differential effect on women, as recently was demonstrated during the COVID-19 pandemic, when far more women than men left the workforce, many due to childcare constraints and widespread school closures.[22] In health care and academics, this may limit women from seeking out or accepting job promotions that come with more responsibilities or greater hours, at the expense of the added income, such as promotions, would bring. Even if no reluctance exists, others in the workplace may assume, for example, that a new mother would not want to take a promotion, which required more hours away from her baby. This perceived reluctance to take on advancement opportunities may be well intentioned on the part of supervisors and bosses, but it serves to limit women's advancement and financial prospects. If the situation is never discussed, a woman may never even realize that she was considered and passed over for a job based on erroneous assumptions.

Ideally, discussions about career goals and responsibilities outside of work could be had in a frank manner. Unfortunately, discussions of work-life balance in the actual workplace are uncommon if not outright taboo. Ironically, a desire to not discriminate has limited the discussions that some employers can have with women about their family lives and reproductive plans. This might prevent discrimination against women in some cases, but also it might allow for discrimination based on imputed assumptions. An open discussion about these subjects would help all parties to parse actual versus imagined reluctance as well as brainstorm solutions that would allow well-qualified women to advance in the workplace while also honoring family commitments. These types of discussions may not be possible until such a time that social change has made the family roles of men and women more equal or until widespread support for childcare gives women sufficient freedom to plan career goals not dependent on the needs of their children.

Even if women do not curtail their career choices due to family responsibilities, it certainly is possible that inefficiencies could be created by women's expanded family roles. Women who are single parents or with little spousal support could be considered to be working 2 jobs, both the surgical career and the household job. The division of attention and mental energy as well as the increased stress could contribute to decreased work productivity. Missed days of work to care for children or last-minute changes to the work schedule also could influence productivity, even if overall hours worked are the same as for male colleagues.

Finally, women may be more likely than men to take on unpaid job roles, such as education and committee work.[23]

STRATEGIES TO ELIMINATE THE GENDER PAY GAP

Transparency in Compensation

Perhaps the most obvious first step is simply to allow for transparency in what people make. Research studies that have evaluated the gender pay gap have relied on surveys or on large government payor databases. This is a cumbersome and inefficient method of sharing information. Specific, anonymized data about salary relative to position, gender, experience, geographic region, and other factors would make it easy to spot any areas of inequality. It would simplify salary negotiation for job applicants and employers, although employers might lose the ability to hire an individual at a discount. If much of the gender bias that drives pay inequality largely is unintentional or at least unrecognized, uncovering the places where it exists should go a long way toward helping rectify it. There are practical barriers to implementing this, which modern computing technology should be able to overcome. There also is cultural sensitivity about money and a general reluctance for people to talk frankly about how much money they make. This barrier may be more difficult to overcome but not impossible.

Educational Components

Training about gender discrimination and implicit bias also is an important and necessary part of the solution. Because so many gender expectations operate at a subconscious level, learning to recognize them is a prerequisite to changing them. This ultimately is an effort that may benefit women the most, but it should not be viewed as punitive toward men. Relieving the tension that exists when gender bias is present will make the workplace more amenable for all. Gender does not exist in a vacuum either but intersects with race, culture, religion, and sexual orientation. Practical and deliberate efforts to improve the institutional attitude toward individuals of different backgrounds ultimately benefit all members.

Training women to be better negotiators also is important. Much of the discussion around gender bias focuses on systemic factors, but merely eliminating the bias that exists does not better equip women to advocate for themselves in the workplace, particularly in sensitive discussions, such as salary, hours, or parental leave. Practical sessions that help women clarify their needs, advocate for themselves, describe their strengths, and overcome objections can help women better communicate in actual job interviews.

Objective Standards of Evaluation

Institutions should develop objective and concrete rubrics for evaluating employee performance and making promotion decisions. Advancement in academics should be guided by objective measures of achievement. This will provide a process whereby the most qualified individuals will be rewarded and the effect of personal preferences can be avoided or at least minimized. It will be helpful for physicians to know on what criteria they will be evaluated, and the organization as a whole can establish clear goals, which are known to all. Performance reviews should be blinded if at all possible, not only to reduce possible positive or negative bias but also to improve confidence in the process itself.

Recently, a majority of symphony orchestras moved to completely blinded audition processes to select their orchestra members. In addition to placing a screen between the musician and the selection jury, a carpet runner also was placed on the stage floor so that even the sound of women's high-heeled shoes would not be an indicator.[24] Since this change, the number of women and racial minorities selected for professional symphony orchestras has increased measurably. The blinded audition process allows for any bias, even the most subtle and insidious, to be nullified. It has been well-received by musicians, who feel they are receiving a fair evaluation, and by music directors who can verify the integrity of their selections.

Although blinded reviews of medical students, residents, and faculty could be challenging, there still are ways to assure the process is as objective as possible. There also is no reason that reviews of grant applications and journal submissions should not be blinded. An individual on a grant committee or an editorial board does not need to know the gender or the race of the person whose work they are evaluating.

SUMMARY

Gender pay inequality is pervasive across professions, including in medicine and surgery. The gap between men and women's earnings increases over time, and women are less prevalent in academic positions of leadership. The causes of the gender pay gap are multifactorial—a common element is implicit bias in the way women are perceived by supervisors, colleagues, and patients and the way women themselves evaluate and navigate career opportunities. Solutions will include efforts at the institutional and specialty levels to recognize bias and counter it as well as hrough increased and transparent reporting of ompensation and objective standards of professional evaluation. Equalizing the gender pay gap s essential for all workers, not only to support authentic collegiality but also so that individual excellence can be celebrated as truly and fairly earned.

DISCLOSURE

The author has nothing to disclose.

REFERENCES

1. American Association of Medical Colleges. Distribution of U.S. medical school faculty by sex, rank, and department. Available at: https://www.aamc.org/download/169810/data/10table13.pdf. Accessed April 30, 2021.

2. Jagsi R, Guancial EA, Worobey CC, et al. The "gender gap" in authorship of academic medical literature—a 35-year perspective. N Engl J Med 2006;355:281–7.

3. Calculation based on data from U.S. Census Bureau, "Current Population Survey: PINC-05. Work Experience-People 15 years of age and Over, by Total Money Earnings, Age, Race, Hispanic Origin, Sex, and Disability Status: 2018". Available at: https://www.census.gov/data/tables/time-series/demo/income-poverty/cps-pinc/pinc-05.html. Accessed April 30, 2021.

4. Langwell KM. Factors affecting the incomes of men and women physicians: further explorations. J Hum Resour 1982;17:261–74.

5. Kehrer BH. Factors affecting the incomes of men and women physicians: An exploratory analysis. J Hum Resour 1976;11:526–45.

6. Ohsfeldt RL, Culler SD. Difference in income between male and female physicians. J Health Econ 1986;5:335–46.

7. Jena AB, Olenski AR, Blumenthal DM. Sex differences in physician salary in us public medical schools. JAMA Intern Med 2016;175:1294–304.

8. Jagsi R, Griffith KA, Stewart A, et al. Gender differences in the salaries of physician researchers. JAMA 2012;307:2410–7.

9. Desai T, Ali S, Fang X, et al. Equal work for unequal pay: the gender reimbursement gap for healthcare providers in the United States. Postgrad Med J 2016;92:571–5.

10. Esteves-Sorenson C, Snyder J. The gender earnings gap for physicians and its increase over time. Econ Lett 2012;116:37–41.

11. Jena AB, Khullar D, Ho O, et al. Sex differences in academic rank in us medical schools in 2014. JAMA 2015;314:1149–58.

12. Arrizabalaga P, Abellana R, Merino A, et al. Gender inequalities in the medical profession: are there still barriers to women physicians in the 21st century? Gac Sanit 2014;28(5):363–8.

13. Association of American Medical Colleges. Physician specialty data report 2016. Available at: https://www.aamc.org/data-reports/workforce/report/physician-specialty-data-report. Accessed April 30, 2021.

14. Riska E. Gender and medical careers. Maturitas 2011;68:264–7.

15. Barbaria P, Abedin S, Berg D, et al. "I'm too used to it": A longitudinal qualitative study of third year female medical students' experience of gendered encounters in medical education. Social Sci Med 2012;74:1013–20.

16. Cochran A, Hauschild T, Elder WB, et al. Perceived gender-based barriers to careers in academic surgery. Am J Surg 2013;206:263–8.

17. Longo P, Straehley CJ. Whack! I've hit the glass ceiling! Women's efforts to gain status in surgery. Gend Med 2008;5:88–100.

18. Webster F, Rice K, Christian J, et al. The erasure of gender in academic surgery: a qualitative study. Am J Surg 2016;212:559–65.

19. Greenberg CC. Association for Academic Surgery presidential address: stick floors and glass ceilings. J Surg Res 2017;219:ix–xviii.

20. Valian V. Why so slow? Cambridge (MA): MIT Press; 1999.

21. Wallis C, Ravi B, Coburn N, et al. Comparison of postoperative outcomes among patients treated by male and female surgeons: a population based matched cohort study. BMJ 2017;359:j4366.

22. Alon T, Doepke M, Olmstead-Rumsey J, et al. The impact of COVID-19 on gender equality. National Bureau of Economic Research; 2020. working paper 26947.

23. Spencer ES, Deal AM, Pruthi NR, et al. Gender differences in compensation, job satisfaction, and other practice patterns in Urology. J Urol 2016;195:450–5.

24. Goldin C, Rouse C. Orchestrating impartiality. The impact of "blind" auditions on female musicians. Am Econ Rev 2000;90:715–41.

Developing a Research Career

Andrea B. Burke, DMD, MD

KEYWORDS

- Surgeon-scientist • Surgical research • Education • Funding • Mentorship
- Career development award

KEY POINTS

- Training the next generation of researchers is critical for the future of oral and maxillofacial surgery.
- Barriers for the surgeon-scientist include the increased demand for clinical productivity, the competitive funding environment, and the struggle to maintain work-life balance.
- Diversity is imperative to build and maintain the next generation of oral and maxillofacial surgery trainees.

INTRODUCTION

Surgeons make excellent scientists thanks to their ability to translate pathophysiology back and forth between the laboratory and the operating room. A surgeon-scientist is in the unique position to contribute to translational research, in the understanding of illness as well as in the development of novel techniques and therapies.[1] Biomedical research is imperative to the future of oral and maxillofacial surgery (OMS) in order to address issues related to diagnosis, disease prevention, and treatment. Research allows us to ask important questions while trying to create better standards of care and improve patient outcomes.

TRAINING SURGEON-SCIENTISTS

A research career must begin with a solid foundation that includes adequate scientific training in addition to surgical education. Structured research training is crucial to the future of all surgical fields, expanding the knowledgebase of trainees while providing an opportunity to train the next generation of academic surgeons.[2,3]

Multiple training models exist: predoctoral training during dental or medical school, dedicated nonclinical time during residency, or a postdoctoral fellowship following clinical training. Ideally,

being exposed to research interests at a young stage in one's career will cultivate future experience. Predoctoral students in college and high school are increasingly exposed to biomedical research in dentistry and medicine. In a study examining compulsory research education in dentistry, Van der Groen and colleagues[4] reported that 74% of students stated that research had a positive impact on their dental education, with a majority (82%) stating that they would remain involved in dental research during their future careers.

Academic surgeons in other fields dispute when research training should be undertaken, with some feeling that it is best to occur in the middle of training, and others who think that it should be done at the conclusion of residency.[5] The Basic Science Committee of the Society of University of Surgeons concluded that a 2-year research training period can provide the fundamental skills necessary to succeed as a surgeon-scientist.[3] Current evidence shows that formal research training is associated with increased scientific productivity and likelihood of future funding through the National Institutes of Health (NIH).[6] Such formal research training during residency has been correlated with higher publication rates as a resident, higher publication impact as a faculty,

The author has nothing to disclose.
Department of Oral & Maxillofacial Surgery, University of Washington School of Dentistry, 1959 Northeast Pacific Street, Box 357134, Seattle, WA 98195-7134, USA
E-mail address: abburke@uw.edu

Oral Maxillofacial Surg Clin N Am 33 (2021) 457–465
https://doi.org/10.1016/j.coms.2021.05.005

and greater chance of having a successful career in academic surgery.[7–9]

Orthopedic surgeons have found controversy in the incorporation of formal research training into residency training.[10] Unsurprisingly, those residents interested in academia found favor in programs with a research track or clinician-scientist training program (T32 grant support through the NIH). They concluded that residency programs with protected research time are helpful with regard to research pursuits but questioned whether all research-track applicants should be interested in academia, given the limited time, mentorship pool, and funding.[10]

Completing a masters or doctoral degree during residency can provide additional educational benefit but comes with the cost of additional training time and financial burden. Alternative approaches include research training during dental or medical school, such as a DDS/DMD or MD-PhD dual-degree program, or for the junior surgeon-scientist to perform a postdoctoral research fellowship following the completion of clinical training. It remains notable that PhDs and dual-degree clinicians receive greater NIH R01 funding than MD or DDS/DMD awardees.[11,12]

Irrespective of when the research is performed, all models must include an appropriate environment and mentor, which will allow the trainee to complete their project in the allotted time. Formal training builds a repertoire of research skills, starting with the ability to generate hypotheses, formulate research questions, and address gaps in knowledge. Taking the time to learn research methodology and various techniques, be they clinical or laboratory, will set the stage for a fruitful career. Projects must be geared toward the strengths of the trainee, while enabling them to develop scholarship skills, including presentation of results and preparation of manuscripts. Finally, the importance of grant-writing skills cannot be stressed enough, along with an understanding of various funding mechanisms for research.[3]

As with any career choice, the decision to train as a surgeon-scientist has its shortcomings. Despite the interest in OMS, the burden of debt from dental and/or medical school may preclude the pursuit of research during or after residency. OMS already requires between 4 and 6 years of postgraduate training, not including fellowship. Added time to an already lengthy training program is one commonly cited downside. Although some clinical research projects can be completed in a short period, 2 years is the minimum that one would need to complete a translational project. For those who choose to pursue additional education, the downside of a dual degree for surgeons is the long gap between completion of research training and the start of the first research job.[2] Furthermore, a postdoctoral fellowship during residency or fellowship might keep up research proficiencies, but at a cost to clinical skills.

Another difficulty is the lack of formal curriculum for research, as most surgical training takes place in a dogmatic atmosphere. Thus, the lack of oversight during research training can be a challenge, as it requires a new way of thinking. Residency accreditation bodies have not provided standards for research education because no established national curriculum exists. In addition, those interested in a research pathway must acquire further skill sets that include managing personnel, writing manuscripts and grants, and mentoring students and fellows.

Working for a stipend while training can preclude a research career altogether.[3] Once a position has been secured, however, the junior surgeon-scientist may be faced with increasing demands for clinical revenue, which inevitably decreases research time.

Finally, surgeons are generally less successful at obtaining NIH funding when compared with non-surgeons. It has been observed that following completion of clinical and research training, most junior faculty are not prepared to become independent investigators, as they still require significant training, mentoring, and support.[5]

ESSENTIALS OF A RESEARCH CAREER

Several factors are important when deciding on a research pathway, and these are summarized in **Box 1**. First and most important is the research environment, whereby the institution needs to be supportive of research activities. At an academic center, there needs to be a commitment to research, with an infrastructure that provides for successful faculty. Scholarly activity and extramural funding within a department are some of the benchmarks to look for when seeking a research position.[2] Other environmental factors include shared equipment or facilities and research cores for routine services (ie, microscopy, histology, genomics, biostatistics). It is important to identify such resources so that funding is not squandered on capital expenses.

Collaborators and a network of experts are an important part of one's environment, as most clinicians and researchers engage in "team science" nowadays. Such relationships can be seen between oral and maxillofacial surgeons, tissue engineers, material scientists, immunologists, geneticists, bioinformaticians, and pharmacologists, to name a few.[12] Finally, grants management

Box 1
Essentials for a successful research career

Environment

  Supportive institution

  Protected research time

  Assistance in developing a robust clinical practice

  Encouragement of activities that build research skills and new techniques

  Adequate facility requirements, equipment, and support staff

  Start-up funding

Mentorship team

  Experienced investigator with track record of success

  Network of collaborators

  Sponsors

Social support

  Backing of family and friends

  Work-life balance

  Family planning

  Set realistic goals

  Learn to transition to and from clinical duties

Area of focus

  Identify problem of interest

  Perform critical assessment of current literature and become an expert

  Tie research interest together with clinical goals

Apply for funding

Avoid conflicts of interest

personnel within the institution are key to navigating the process from application to disbursement.

Protected research time is another essential component to a successful endeavor because it allows for uninterrupted focus and dedication to research efforts. The proportion of effort is highly dependent on the individual researcher and includes support from the institution, chairperson, and colleagues. It should be noted that this protected time also should include supervising/mentoring trainees and staff, writing papers and grants, and attending conferences.[13] The careful balance between clinical responsibilities and research goals may make or break a young surgeon-scientist. Balancing clinical responsibilities and research goals can become particularly challenging in the beginning of one's surgical career, when more time is dedicated to patient care and establishing oneself. Working as a team with supportive surgeons can help protect a junior surgeon's research time. Moreover, some institutions offer compensation for academic productivity, such as grants, and develop lower relative value unit expectations for those surgeons striving to build their research.[2]

A mentor can be defined as a teacher, adviser, role model, advocate, and friend.[14] As previously mentioned, most young researchers have a mentorship team, making it less critical for a single mentor to possess all these traits. The importance of a healthy mentor relationship cannot be stressed enough and is built on a mutual commitment with shared interests. Foremost, a mentor will help one establish realistic and achievable goals. They will educate and provide advice, motivate and establish collaborations, and assist with challenges, such as negotiating a new position. A good mentor will have a history of successful relationships with mentees who develop into independent investigators. As there are two sides to this relationship, it is key that the mentee be proactive, focused, a good listener, and open to critique. Likewise, sponsorship is a similar association, in which the sponsor leverages their reputation and network to endorse and promote the mentee's career advancement.[15]

Choosing a research area of focus may be within one's specialty or with a supervisor outside the field. Topics such as biomaterials, genomics, tissue engineering, or other technology may require a concentration outside of OMS. Having a basic science mentor in addition to a clinical mentor will help bolster translational research projects from bench to bedside. Moreover, a partnership with nonclinicians can help offset the clinical demands of surgical patient care.

Personal factors are crucial when deciding on a research career. In a survey of 459 general surgery residents, 79% of women and 55% of men felt that the opportunity to take a break from residency was an influential factor for doing research.[15] The concept of work-life balance is the notion that one's self-worth is attached to the sense of self, family, work, and community. Although one's personal life and family life are integral to a career, having too much of one or the other can be seen as a major impediment to success.[1] Combining clinical and scientific endeavors is inevitably going to lead to long hours and frustration, so it is important to develop an institutional culture that supports personal goals while working to prevent burnout. Increased flexibility in work hours and the ability to perform some tasks (ie, data analysis, manuscript preparation) from home may help to maintain balance. Likewise, it is equally important to have a strong social network to support a surgeon-scientist. Setting realistic expectations establishes the context for success at work and in one's personal life.

It is a common conception that a research-focused career is less financially rewarding than a purely clinical pathway. With educational debt and cost of living to consider, an early commitment makes planning a research career more feasible. Negotiating a start-up package is vital when starting out as a junior surgeon-scientist. This package provides essential funds ("seed money") for basics, such as laboratory reagents, shared equipment, key personnel, and salaries, and is fundamental to generating preliminary data in order to apply for future financial support. Physical laboratory space, if necessary, is also a negotiable item, and for the surgeon, proximity to clinical workspace should be considered.

It is also important to understand how compensation is structured, particularly when clinical revenue is considered. The junior surgeon-scientist must understand their funding environment and establish timelines early on. For instance, one must consider stipulations for renewal of start-up funds, resources provided, shared equipment, technical cores, and so forth. Because it is common to have 3 to 5 years before benchmarks are met, funding may need to be extended. The average age for an awardee's first R01 grant is 45 years old.[16] Thus, although the perfect job offer is unlikely, it is imperative to determine what resources will be important for success and make one's wishes known.

Knowledge of the promotions process with regard to research timelines will be of utmost importance in setting goals and maximizing productivity. With extramural funding as the goal, the junior surgeon-scientist should receive support to gain further research education, particularly if they did not have the chance as a trainee. This self-study may require a transition back and forth between clinical duties, as one spends the first few months identifying the scientific questions that will become their area of research focus, rigorously reviewing the current literature and becoming an expert on the topic. Formal coursework, such as biostatistics, clinical research study design, and grant writing, must be a part of research activity and protected time. Learning laboratory protocols, experimental approaches, computer programs, and various techniques may also be required. A career development award through the NIH allows physicians to maintain a clinical practice while attaining these skills and simultaneously developing an area of original scientific investigation. However, the goal should be to convert the career development award into an independently funded research award or an R01.[5]

Finally, conflicts of interest and professional conduct in research are concepts that a surgeon-scientist will be confronted with. Institutional review boards (IRBs) were created to protect human subjects involved in research. Understanding IRB requirements and maintaining research integrity are paramount, whether performing a retrospective chart review or an interventional study.

BARRIERS

Multiple challenges exist in a career as a surgeon-scientist.[2] There has been a 27% proportional decrease in NIH funding to Departments of Surgery, relative to total NIH funding, between 2007 and 2014.[1,2] Such findings, combined with the dwindling numbers of grant applications and research grants awarded to surgeons when compared with their nonsurgeon colleagues, significantly contributes to the attrition of surgeons pursuing a research career.[2,17] Other barriers include the increased demand for clinical productivity and administrative roles, additional regulations on research studies, and the ever present struggle to maintain work-life balance. Protected research time needs to be sacrosanct, as surgeon leaders confront the changing landscape of academia.

The NIH "strongly believes that diversity in the biomedical research workforce is critical to producing new scientific discoveries."[18] An NIH-sponsored study was created to ascertain the disparity in R01 grant funding to African American applicants. As a result, the first Chief Officer for Scientific Workforce Diversity and an Advisory Committee to the Director's Working Group on Diversity in the Biomedical Research Workforce were created. One long-term goal was the BUILD Initiative (BUilding Infrastructure Leading to Diversity), which seeks to create cultural changes at academic institutions so that historically underrepresented groups in biomedical research could prepare for research careers. In addition, the NIH National Research Mentoring Network pairs underrepresented groups across the country with researchers to build the workforce. OMS must make diversity a top priority, capitalizing on unique perspectives and recruiting talented trainees.

Some of the deterrents that dissuade underrepresented groups, including women, from entering research fields include the stress of competition with regard to grants, financial instability of projects, and the perceived isolation of scientific research.[19] Studies have shown that interest in research and experiential learning motivates students, and the right mentor can influence research-career decisions. Pipeline programs are excellent strategies to encourage and support underrepresented groups and develop retention from a young age. Programs that include research experiences report improved academics, self-efficacy, and positive attitudes.[19] Thus, it is not enough to improve the diversity of the clinical and translational research workforce; protocols must be implemented to retain members of underrepresented groups throughout their biomedical research careers.

Women remain underrepresented in academic surgery.[20] Consequently, there are inadequate numbers of female role models and mentors for women in surgery. This paucity of female mentors is evidenced by the persistent gender gap at senior levels of academia, where women are less likely to become full professors across surgical fields, even when factors such as age, years in practice, publication record, NIH funding, and other factors are controlled. It should also be noted that home and childcare responsibilities, even in surgery, still disproportionately fall to women and that pregnancies and/or parental leaves often coincide with an age when career advancement most often occurs.[21]

Progressively, institutions are making efforts to improve gender equality in academic medicine by understanding the barriers that face junior physician-faculty researchers.[22] It is concerning that the surgeon-scientist track has shown that less than 50% of NIH K-series career development awards went on to achieve R01 independent awards, with women performing worse than men.[23] In evaluating K08 and K23 mentored career development awards, Jagsi and colleagues[22,23] found that men and women have different experiences at work and at home, with respect to career outcomes and academic success. As an example, protected research time appeared more important for the success of female clinician-scientists, leading them to advocate for practices that increase a woman's ability to access and spend time on research.

Success in research can take many forms but is generally seen as obtaining extramural funding and publication in high-impact journals. There remains no uniform metric for success as a surgeon-scientist, and there is a discrepancy between the elements that comprise a successful research career. Women are more likely to emphasize objective measures (such as publications) and relational skills (such as networking and collaboration), as compared with men, who emphasize boldness, critical thinking, and confidence.[24]

RESEARCH CAREER OPPORTUNITIES

Research disciplines can generally be broken into basic science and translational and clinical research, with surgeon-scientists participating in all phases. Basic science research typically occurs in the laboratory setting and focuses on the human bodily functions as they relate to health and disease. Studies can range from cellular and molecular to physiologic mechanisms and systems biology. Basic research provides the foundation of knowledge for applied or translational research, better known as "bench to bedside." Translational research can take the form of clinical, preclinical, or animal experiments, with the goal of applying basic research to human models. Often, translational therapies build on basic research to create new diagnostics, techniques, and therapies **(Fig. 1)**. Surgeon-scientists are at the forefront of translational medicine, with accessibility to tissue specimens and the ability to perform novel techniques. Finally, clinical research focuses on disease diagnosis, prevention, and treatment in order to retrospectively examine trends, apply evidence-based medicine, develop clinical trials,

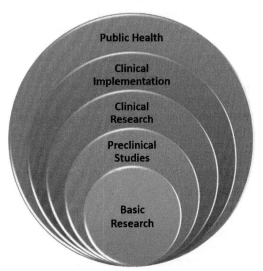

Fig. 1. Stages of research. Each stage builds on and informs the others, starting with the fundamental mechanisms of disease at the basic level, extending to model interventions in preclinical studies (ie, cellular or animal models), to human interventions. Clinical research aims to understand disease as it relates to such models, testing for outcomes and reporting on safety and effectiveness. Clinical implementation research disseminates the results of clinical trials and identifies gaps in care. Finally, public health studies the outcomes at the population level to determine the effects of diseases, while working to diagnose, prevent and treat.

and extrapolate population-based studies. The gold standard of clinical research remains the randomized clinical trial, which seeks to improve patient outcomes. Other research endeavors may include public policy, education, bioinformatics, and data science, to name a few.

A research career in OMS can prove to be a gratifying alternative career path, which can take many forms. In addition to academia, there are a multitude of career opportunities in the public and private sectors. Federal agencies, such as the Food and Drug Administration, the Centers for Disease Control and Prevention, and the NIH, are major research centers that employ clinician-scientists. The military, including the Department of Veterans Affairs system, also has positions for oral and maxillofacial surgeons, with the prospect of conducting research.[12] The American Dental Association Foundation, located at the National Institute of Standards and Technology, is another national organization with career opportunities geared toward dentists and maxillofacial surgeons. Another such example is the Agency for Healthcare Research and Quality, tasked with improving safety standards and informing policy related to the United States' health care system.

The NIH, and specifically the National Institute of Dental and Craniofacial Research (NIDCR), has multiple training programs available to those interested in research at all career stages. The Dental Summer Research Internship is an intensive summer program providing current dental students with a small taste of research experience. The Medical Research Scholars Program is a 1-year research fellowship for dental and medical students. The NIDCR Clinical Research Fellowship is a research mechanism for trainees who have completed doctoral training and are interested in pursuing a research career. Finally, the NIH has numerous opportunities for postdoctoral research fellowships.

For others, a research career based in industry may provide financial freedoms and job flexibility. Medical device companies, the defense sector, and pharmaceutical industries are just a few private-sector opportunities available to oral and maxillofacial surgeons. Projects with a product-driven mission will benefit from the perspective of surgeon-scientists who can assist with development.

FUNDING MECHANISMS

Funding is necessary to support research activities and can be quite competitive to obtain. Therefore, grant-writing is pivotal to the success of the surgeon-scientist. The NIH has numerous mechanisms to fund research during all phases of one's career: Predoctoral and postdoctoral awards (F) support dual-degree programs and research-tracks during training, respectively. In addition, the NIH has the Loan Repayment Program (www.lrp.nih.gov/) available to clinical investigators engaged in research.

As previously mentioned, mentored career development (K) and independent research project grants (R) are among those awards that fund early- and late-stage investigators. Typically, early career physician-scientists must develop an aptitude in basic or translational research, and independence is expected to take 5 years when transitioning from a K-award to an R-award. **Table 1** lists the major NIH career development awards available. The application process can be arduous, taking 20 months on average. Further complicating matters is the issue of protected time as a junior surgeon; the K-awards are excellent because they protect 75% of the research effort, but some institutions may not be able to support this much time away from clinical duties. In some instances, the time commitment for K-awards has been reduced to 50% for surgeons as a special exception. Developing a relationship with NIH program officers in the Office of Extramural Research is key to grant success.

Given the challenges with extramural funding through the NIH, young investigators may consider grant mechanisms through departments, hospitals or institutions, private foundations, and specialty societies. Specific to OMS, the American Association of Oral and Maxillofacial Surgeons created the Faculty Educator Development Award to promote academic recruitment and retention. These grants were developed to offset the financial burdens of an academic career by providing funds that go directly to the awardee. In addition, the Oral and Maxillofacial Surgery Foundation offers research support grants and student research training awards (http://omsfoundation.org). Other specialty organizations that provide funding include the OsteoScience Foundation (www.osteoscience.org/), AO Foundation (https://aocmf.aofoundation.org/), and the American Cleft Palate-Craniofacial Association (www.acpa-cpf.org/). National funding bodies, such as The National Science Foundation and the Defense Advanced Research Projects Agency (www.darpa.mil/), provide endowments to a variety of research areas that may overlap with surgical fields, including engineering, environmental research, and social sciences. Finally, charitable organizations, patient advocacy groups, and industry sponsors may provide additional means for private research funds. Some private

Table 1
Major National Institutes of Health career development awards designed for individual researchers (basic science and clinical)

Program	Description
K08	Mentored Clinical Scientist Carter Development Award • Designed for physician-scientists and PhDs with clinical appointments • Primarily dedicated to research not involving human subjects • Largest source of career development support to individual researchers • Provides 3–5 y of grant support; requires 75% dedicated effort • Supported by all major NIH institutes
K01	Mentored Research Scientist Career Development Award • Designed primarily for nonclinician career researchers (junior faculty-level PhDs) • Provides 3–5 y of grant support; requires 75% dedicated effort • Supported by most NIH institutes
K07	Academic Career Development Award • Designed to foster leadership roles for academicians (clinical and nonclinical faculty) interested in expanding an institution's expertise in a given field or area of research • Provides 2–5 y of grant support: requires 75% dedicated effort • Sponsorship is limited to few NIH institutes (NIA, NIAAA, NCI, NIMH, NCCAM)
K23	Mentored Patient-Oriented Research Career Development Award • Designed for physician-scientists with clinical appointments (junior faculty-level MDs) • Specifically dedicated to career development in patient-oriented research • Provides 3–5 y of grant support; requires 75% dedicated effort • Program widely implemented in 1999; sponsored by most NIH institutes
K24	Mid-Career Investigator Award in Patient-Oriented Research • Designed to support established clinical researchers (senior faculty-level MDs) who are interested in developing a mentorship infrastructure for young clinical investigators • Provides 3–5 y of grant support; requires 25% to 50% dedicated effort • Program widely implemented in 1999; sponsored by most NIH institutes

From Rangel SJ, Moss RL. Recent trends in the funding and utilization of NIH career development awards by surgical faculty. Surgery 2004;136(2):232-239; with permission.

organizations are The American Cancer Society, Arthritis Foundation, Robert Wood Johnson Foundation, Doris Duke Charitable Foundation, and the Burroughs Wellcome Fund.[5]

SUMMARY

Research is critical for the future of OMS, as the understanding of diseases and treatments evolves. Unfortunately, in the current environment, there are too few physician-scientists to replace those who are retiring. Leaders of departments and institutions must recognize the pressure and time constraints that are being imposed by increased demands for clinical revenue from young faculty. Organizations must be proactive to alleviate such pressures, protecting young investigators and facilitating an environment that allows them to develop into independent investigators. Furthermore, building diverse teams of surgeon-scientists from underrepresented groups is imperative in order to mentor the next generation of trainees.

A research career in OMS can provide the variety, flexibility, and fulfillment that many of us seek. The surgeon-scientist must possess a passion for research and be persistent and resilient. Developing a supportive social network and mentorship team will help pave the road to success. Although there may be many pitfalls and failures along the way, scientific thinking and research skills will have a positive impact on clinical practice. Ultimately, whether one chooses to publish a case report or develop a clinical trial, everyone can participate in research at any stage of their career.

REFERENCES

1. Keswani SG, Moles CM, Morowitz M, et al. The future of basic science in academic surgery: identifying barriers to success for surgeon-scientists. Ann Surg 2017;265(6):1053–9.
2. Goldstein AM, Blair AB, Keswani SG, et al. A roadmap for aspiring surgeon-scientists in today's healthcare environment. Ann Surg 2019;269(1): 66–72.
3. Zuo KJ, Meng Y, Gordon L, et al. Navigating the postgraduate research fellowship: a roadmap for surgical residents. J Surg Res 2020;256:282–9.
4. Van der Groen TA, Olsen BR, Park SE. Effects of a research requirement for dental students: a retrospective analysis of students' perspectives across ten years. J Dent Educ 2018;82(11):1171–7.
5. Suliburk JW, Kao LS, Kozar RA, et al. Training future surgical scientists: realities and recommendations. Ann Surg 2008;247(5):741–9.
6. Lopez J, Ameri A, Susarla SM, et al. Does formal research training lead to academic success in plastic surgery? A comprehensive analysis of U.S. academic plastic surgeons. J Surg Educ 2016;73(3): 422–8.
7. Andriole DA, Klingensmith ME, Fields RC, et al. Is dedicated research time during surgery residency associated with surgeons' future career paths?: a national study. Ann Surg 2020;271(3):590–7.
8. Ellis MC, Dhungel B, Weerasinghe R, et al. Trends in research time, fellowship training, and practice patterns among general surgery graduates. J Surg Educ 2011;68(4):309–12.
9. Hsieh H, Paquette F, Fraser SA, et al. Formal research training during surgical residency: scaffolding for academic success. Am J Surg 2014; 207(1):141–5.
10. Mittwede PN, Morales-Restrepo A, Fourman MS, et al. Research-track residency programs in orthopaedic surgery: a survey of program directors and recent graduates. J Bone Joint Surg Am 2019; 101(15):1420–7.
11. Thompson DF. Understanding financial conflicts of interest. N Engl J Med 1993;329(8):573–6.
12. Fonseca RJ, DMD. Oral & maxillofacial surgery. 3rd edition. Philadelphia: Saunders (Elsevier); 2017.
13. Tai IT. Developing a clinician-scientist career. Clin Invest Med 2008;31(5):E300–1.
14. Brock MV, Bouvet M. Writing a successful NIH Mentored Career Development Grant (K award): hints for the junior faculty surgeon. Ann Surg 2010;251(6): 1013–7.
15. Ayyala MS, Skarupski K, Bodurtha JN, et al. Mentorship is not enough: exploring sponsorship and its role in career advancement in academic medicine. Acad Med 2019;94(1):94–100.
16. Garrison HH, Deschamps AM. NIH research funding and early career physician scientists: continuing challenges in the 21st century. FASEB J 2014; 28(3):1049–58.
17. Rangel SJ, Moss RL. Recent trends in the funding and utilization of NIH career development awards by surgical faculty. Surgery 2004;136(2): 232–9.
18. NIH-Wide Strategic Plan: Fiscal years 2016-2020. Available at: https://www.nih.gov/sites/default/files/about-nih/strategic-plan-fy2016-2020-508.pdf.
19. Bhatt R, West B, Chaudhary S. Biomedical career enrichment programs: exploring women and minority participants' motivators and outcomes. PLoS One 2020;15(2):e0228934.
20. Zhuge Y, Kaufman J, Simeone DM, et al. Is there still a glass ceiling for women in academic surgery? Ann Surg 2011;253(4):637–43.
21. Tulunay-Ugur OE, Sinclair CF, Chen AY. Assessment of gender differences in perceptions of work-life integration among head and neck

surgeons. JAMA Otolaryngol Head Neck Surg 2019;145(5):453–8.

22. Jagsi R, Griffith KA, Jones RD, et al. Factors associated with success of clinician-researchers receiving career development awards from the National Institutes of Health: a longitudinal cohort study. Acad Med 2017;92(10):1429–39.

23. Jagsi R, Motomura AR, Griffith KA, et al. Sex differences in attainment of independent funding by career development awardees. Ann Intern Med 2009;151(11):804–11.

24. Gotian R, Andersen OS. How perceptions of a successful physician-scientist varies with gender and academic rank: toward defining physician-scientist's success. BMC Med Educ 2020;20(1):50.

Work–Life Balance for Oral and Maxillofacial Surgeons

Sara Hinds Anderson, MS, DDS, MD[a], Justine Sherylyn Moe, MD, DDS[a],
Shelly Abramowicz, DMD, MPH, FACS[b],*

KEYWORDS

• Work–life balance • Work–life integration • Burnout • Work–life conflict • Mindfulness • Resilience

KEY POINTS

• Work–life integration, in contrast with work–life balance, offers an achievable goal; an oral and maxillofacial surgeon's personal and professional lives are aligned to improve overall satisfaction, performance, and efficiency.
• Work–life integration can be optimized by appraising one's current distribution of time and focus on the 4 life domains while identifying gaps in this distribution compared with desired individual goals.
• Burnout is one's response to ongoing stress, marked by cynicism, depersonalization, detachment and lack of sense of personal accomplishment, which is correlated with mental health issues, medical errors and poor patient outcomes.
• Gender and ethnicity have a complex impact on work–life integration and burnout.
• Strategies on individual and organization levels exist for improved work–life integration to prevent burnout.

INTRODUCTION

Work–life integration in oral and maxillofacial surgery (OMS) training and practice can be challenging, but is important for career satisfaction as well as individual and team performances. Rates of physician burnout are higher than the general population[1]; challenges to work–life integration and surgeon well-being have recently become an emerging area of research. Despite this increased recognition, at the time of this publication, there is a paucity of literature that qualifies, quantifies, and identifies interventions to improve work–life integration to decrease physician burnout.

Four domains have been described in consideration of work–life integration: work, home, community, and self.[2] The commonly used term work–life balance is suggestive of mandatory trade-offs among various domains. The term work–life integration offers a more pragmatic goal in the pursuit of personal and professional gains. Therefore, the authors use the term work–life integration for the remainder of this article. Work–life integration promotes surgeon well-being, which is a complex interplay of physical, emotional, mental, social, and spiritual factors.[3,4] Finding time for the home, community, and self domains, which can often be neglected particularly during surgical training, is critical for preserving and developing mental health and avoiding burnout.[5,6]

Although often viewed through the lens of conflicting priorities, the 4 domains can be integrated with intentionality, for mutual gain by achieving the so-called 4-way win. Once this integration is negotiated, there can be an increase in career satisfaction and performance, often paradoxically while

a Department of Oral and Maxillofacial Surgery, Michigan Medicine, 1500 East Medical Center Drive, Ann Arbor, MI 48109, USA; b Division of Oral and Maxillofacial Surgery, Department of Surgery, Emory University School of Medicine, 1365 Clifton Road, Building B, Suite 2300, Atlanta, GA 30322, USA
* Corresponding author.
E-mail address: sabram5@emory.edu

Oral Maxillofacial Surg Clin N Am 33 (2021) 467–473
https://doi.org/10.1016/j.coms.2021.05.006

working fewer hours and allocating more energy and focus outside of the work domain.[2] The proportion of time and attention devoted to the 4 domains varies between individuals. Establishing boundaries between each domain's competing demands requires preemptive consideration of personal priorities. In his book *Total Leadership: Be a Better Leader, Have a Richer Life*,[7] Stewart Friedman describes an assessment tool that can be used to uncover discrepancies in assigned importance and focused energy as well as personal satisfaction (**Box 1**).

It is important to take the time to define personal priorities. Compromise between domains is inevitable and should be embraced not as a failure, but as successful negotiations. It is helpful to remember that small and realistic changes can create incredible benefits for surgeons. An increase in efficiency, focus, and productivity allows a greater sense of fulfillment and satisfaction.

WORK–LIFE INTEGRATION IN ORAL AND MAXILLOFACIAL SURGERY

An individual who chooses the discipline of OMS is typically driven and ambitious and places a high emphasis on achievement.[8] While working long hours, OMS surgeons make innumerable sacrifices for their patients and practice. It would be remiss to not acknowledge that this drive is central to the promotion and progression of the profession. The authors of this article believe that this achievement should not be at the expense of the surgeon's health and self-fulfillment.

A recent survey of 2295 retired general surgeons aimed to evaluate reflections on their lives and careers.[9] The most common regret reported (61.8%) was wishing they could have achieved a better work–life integration during their career.[9] Other self-reported wishes included making more time for family and personal wellness or joining a less stressful practice environment. Only 1.1% wished they had made more money; this finding is consistent with prior studies demonstrating a 2% correlation between salary and career satisfaction.[2,9] This survey challenges the historical stereotype of surgeons[10,11] with regard to work–life integration and sheds light on potentially modifiable factors that could augment the careers of surgeons.

When overimportance is placed on a single life domain, the others tend to suffer as a result and this creates personal disharmony, which can have significant physical and psychological health consequences. Furthermore, surgeons may incorrectly believe that, by neglecting our other life domains, we will be more successful in the work

domain; however, this supposition is not necessarily true and often unsustainable.[2]

WORK–LIFE CONFLICT AND BURNOUT

Burnout is closely associated with poor work–life integration and many of the same factors contribute to both.[12] A career in surgery can be both highly rewarding and highly stressful. Throughout the course of a surgeon's career from trainee to practitioner, innumerable challenges will present themselves that can lead to distress and dissatisfaction despite the many virtues of the surgical profession.

In a recent survey of 7197 general surgeons, 52% reported experiencing work–home conflict in the last 3 weeks,[13] which demonstrates the high strain that surgeon's careers typically place on their personal lives. Furthermore, this study showed that surgeons who experience work–home conflict were significantly more likely to experience burnout.[13] Work–home conflicts were also independently associated with an increased likelihood of decreased clinical work hours or a plan to leave current practice, which has implications for the retention of talented surgeons in the workforce.

National averages for burnout and depression among surgeons (including OMS) are alarmingly high.[1,14] Burnout is a syndrome of work-related stress and emotional exhaustion. Symptoms of burnout include cynicism, depersonalization, detachment, and a lack of a sense of personal accomplishment.[15] Physicians and surgeons who suffer from burnout often report feeling unfulfilled and disconnected from their patients and have a diminished sense of personal accomplishment.[6,15]

A cross-sectional survey of members of the American College of Surgeons revealed that 40% of responding surgeons were burned out and 30% screened positive for symptoms of depression.[16] Factors independently associated with burnout included younger age, having children, area of specialization, number of nights on call per week, hours worked per week, and having compensation determined entirely based on billing.

Major contributors to burnout include the increasing burden of bureaucratic tasks and computerization of practice on surgeons and medical providers.[1] Overtime, these tasks erode the surgeons well-being and create a phenomenon of depersonalization.[1,17]

Burnout occurs most often for physicians who are mid-career, but also peaks during residency.[1,14] Surgical residency is an intense time of sacrifice and commitment that is imperative

Box 1
Work–life integration assessment tool

a. On a percentage basis, how important is each one of the 4 domains to you now?

Domain	Importance
Work, career	_____%
Home, family	_____%
Community, society	_____%
Self: body, mind, spirit	_____%
Total	100%

b. On a percentage basis, how much do you focus your attention on each of the 4 domains in a typical week or month?

Domain	Focus of Time and Energy
Work, career	_____%
Home, family	_____%
Community, society	_____%
Self: body, mind, spirit	_____%
Total	100%

c. How satisfied are you in each of the 4 domains?

Domain	Not Satisfied		Fully Satisfied
Work, career	1	2 3 4 5 6	7 8 9 10
Home, family	1	2 3 4 5 6	7 8 9 10
Community, society	1	2 3 4 5 6	7 8 9 10
Self: body, mind, spirit	1	2 3 4 5 6	7 8 9 10

From Friedman SD, Saunders EG, Bregman P and Dowling D. Chapter 2: Assessment: Are You Focusing on What's Important to You? In: HBR Guide to Work–Life Balance. Harvard Business Publishing, 2019. 34-35; with permission.

residents, 51% suffer from moderate to severe emotional exhaustion and 85.7% suffer from moderate to severe depersonalization, which can contribute to higher levels of medical errors.[14,18] This study also assessed the effects of shame on resident well-being and burnout, finding a reported incidence of 70% of residents experiencing shaming events during their residency, most commonly in the operating room. Those who were perpetually shamed were more likely to suffer depression, burnout and poor job performance.[14] A separate study of OMS residents showed that dissatisfaction was associated with higher stress scores.[5]

The trend toward dramatically high levels of burnout is particularly concerning when patient safety is examined. Major medical errors have been shown to be associated with higher levels of burnout and mental health issues among American surgeons.[18] A medical error is a preventable mistake made by a provider with potentially adverse outcomes and is distinct from a surgical complication, which is an adverse outcome that is an acknowledged and known risk of the procedure. Using standardized assessment tools, a recent study demonstrated that burnout and depression are both independent predictors for reporting major events with an odds ratio 2.0 and 2.2, respectively, on multivariate analysis. In fact, for each point increase in depersonalization (on a validated scale of 0–33) there is an 11% increase in the likelihood of reporting an error. From a patient safety standpoint, there should be an emphasis on creating strategies that decrease surgeon burnout.

In addition to higher levels of depression, physicians are also at high risk for attempting and committing suicide. An estimated 300 to 400 physicians commit suicide per year.[1] Within that context, decreasing the emotional exhaustion and burnout of physicians with a greater emphasis on work–life integration is not an indulgence, but a necessity.

GENDER AND WORK–LIFE INTEGRATION

Over the last few decades, there has been an increase in the proportion of women in surgery and OMS as a subset, albeit at a disproportionately slower rate.[19–21] Although men and women alike struggle with work–life integration during their careers, gender has been shown to play a significant role in the way that balance is achieved. For women, the challenge of managing the 4 domains (work, home, community, and self) can be particularly difficult, in part because women tend to juggle more roles and are more likely to be primarily

for fostering competent and knowledgeable surgeons. This is a high-risk time for burnout, and therefore research is needed to identify potentially modifiable risk factors for targeted intervention. Residents tend to report high stress levels, which can precipitate burnout as well as mental and physical health issues.[6] A cross-sectional study of 566 surgical residents demonstrated a 69% prevalence rate of burnout.[6] The same study showed that higher levels of stress correlated with burnout and dispositional mindfulness was associated with lower rates of burnout.

Specifically within OMS, residents are also struggling with the effects of stress and burnout. In a cross-sectional analysis of 217 OMS responsible for organizing the home.[22,23] Dual professional partnerships are very common. In a survey of academic surgeons, 97% of female surgeons reported being married to another professional, compared with 37% for their male counterparts. Of the married female surgeons, 100% of their partners worked full time.[23] Within their marriages, women reported being more likely to be responsible for organizing childcare, meal planning, grocery shopping, and vacation planning. Women are also more likely to experience work–home conflict compared with men and often their conflicts stem from their partner's career.[24] In a recent survey, the majority of female OMS residents were satisfied with OMS; however, they had less job satisfaction when compared with their male counterparts.[25] This observed gender difference does not persist in academic OMS surgeons and private practitioners.

Regarding gender differences in family planning, men during residency are more likely to be married (91.0% vs 75.6%) and have children (91.3% vs 63.8%) with a reported two-thirds of female residents intentionally choosing to delay childbirth.[26] Although the cause of this is likely multifactorial, there are many perceived barriers and pressures that female residents face to avoid maternity during residency. Women surgeons are more likely to believe that child-rearing slowed their career advancement, although notably the same study found no difference in the number of hours worked and nights on call per week between men and women.[24] Given what is already known about work–life conflict and burnout, it is not surprising that more women than men surgeons had burnout and depressive symptoms.[5,24] Policies that offer protection for women who opt for child-birth and child rearing during residency would be beneficial in the recruitment and retention of promising female applicants.[27,28]

ETHNICITY AND WORK–LIFE INTEGRATION

Previous research demonstrated associations between gender, work–life integration, and burnout. However, the role of race/ethnicity is not well-understood. Physicians in minority racial/ethnic groups have been shown to have experiences that might negatively affect work–life integration (ie, social isolation, discrimination by colleagues and patients, and more frequent delegation of nonclinical tasks associated with the promotion of workplace diversity and inclusion).[29–31]

A cross-sectional national study of 4424 physicians[31] found that Hispanic/Latino, non-Hispanic Black, and non-Hispanic Asian physicians reported lower rates of occupational burnout compared with non-Hispanic White physicians. The odds of burnout are lowest among Black physicians and highest among White physicians. Black physicians were more likely to be satisfied with work–life integration compared with White physicians, and there were no differences by race/ethnicity observed for depressive symptoms or career satisfaction.

Multiple studies addressing the effect of race/ethnicity on burnout among medical trainees have found varying results.[32–34] Additional studies are required to further comprehend the nature of these perceptions, including the possible role of early attrition of minority racial/ethnic groups from medicine during training, the effect of race/ethnicity on the willingness to disclose burnout symptoms, and the role of life experience of minority racial/ethnic groups in promoting resilience.[35]

Within OMS, the racial demographic of OMS practitioners does not match the racial demographic of the United States.[36] A survey of 41 African American OMS[37] found that a significant proportion experienced race-related harassment (25%–46%) and bias (48%–55%). However, these events did not seem to affect professional success; most respondents reported no effect on application to residency and success of their practice. Much work needs to be done to understand the impact of ethnicity on work–life integration within OMS.

STRATEGIES FOR WORK–LIFE INTEGRATION

Given the prevalence and severity of burnout and mental health issues among physicians and surgeons, there has recently been an effort toward developing strategies to promote improved work–life integration. These strategies can be grouped into individual and organizational initiatives.

On the individual level, surgeons can work toward establishing better work–life integration by evaluating their personal values regarding the 4 life domains.[2] By acknowledging that time and energy are finite, surgeons can learn to refocus and reset their priorities to become better surgeons, family members, and members of their community. Articulating personal needs and values, for example, with the assessment tool in **Box 1**, is the first step toward identifying desynchrony and imbalance.[2]

Recently there has been a growing interest in customizing career paths that incorporate flexibility to facilitate work–life integration; these new models are not restricted by outdated career rules that are not aligned with personal and cultural value system.[2] Negotiation skills, which are not traditionally taught in medical training, are an important component of the medical business and can be used by surgeons to optimize and customize their careers.[38,39] There is currently a dearth of research with regard to contract negotiation and work–life integration in surgery; the authors suggest considering the tradeoff between salary, time commitment, schedule flexibility, clinical support, and dedicated research time. Of note, 49% of physicians report that they would take a pay cut to work better hours and improve their work–life integration.[1]

Individual wellness and resilience have been shown to improve surgeon career satisfaction.[16,40] Resilience is a learned personality trait that determines how well an individual can cope with stress. Resilience enables surgeons to thrive in the face of adversity.[16,40–42] In a survey of OMS residents, those who had coping skills, exercised, and practiced relaxation reported higher levels of overall satisfaction, a surrogate for resident well-being.[5] Additionally, mindfulness tendencies among surgery residents have been shown to be associated with a significantly decreased risk of burnout, anxiety, depression, and suicidal ideation.[6] Mindfulness skills and personal grit can be taught through stress resilience interventions, training and feedback.[6,41,42]

The ability of individuals to modify burnout that is related to the organizational and bureaucratic burden may be limited. System changes and organizational policies are vital to the promotion of work–life integration for surgeons. Studies show that organizational interventions to prevent and mitigate physician burnout are effective.[43,44] Through the STEPS Forward Initiative,[45] the American Medical Association developed a national tool kit to disseminate strategies to recognize and address physician burnout and promote physician well-being through workplace culture. The National Academy of Medicine released a consensus report in 2019[46] exploring the factors and consequences of clinician burnout and providing a framework for a systems approach to clinical burnout and professional well-being by engaging health care organizations, electronic health record providers, private payers, and other critical stakeholders.

Organizational changes to workplace culture can be promoted by a chief wellness officer and a wellness committee.[45,47] The wellness officer and committee are tasked with promoting policies and initiatives that facilitate physical and mental health through education and engagement. The role of this committee can be to establish an environment of psychological safety, provide mental health resources, maintain the educational missions, solidify a sense of community by showing appreciation, and using social media to promote community morale.[47] Among OMS residents, those who reported having access to mental health services had a 6.52 times greater odd of satisfaction compared with those residents who did not have access to those resources.[5] On the department and division levels, leadership qualities have been shown to correlate with department well-being; higher leadership composite ratings among division and department chairs is associated with a lower risk of burnout and higher prevalence of satisfaction,[48] which demonstrates the importance of leadership training for physicians.

Policies that accommodate flexibility for family and medical leave can promote surgeon wellness. OMS residents surveyed who were able to take a family or medical leave of absence had a 3.35 times greater odd of satisfaction among those residents who never received a leave of absence.[5] The American Board of Surgery has a policy for the protection of maternity, paternity, and family leave; however, a survey of general surgery residents showed that this leave was often underused in part owing to a lack of a universal leave policy, strain on the residency program, and the loss of education and training time, as well as a lack of flexibility and perceived support.[49] Improved national and organizational policies that promote family leave will in turn improve the well-being and retention of the surgical workforce.[28]

SUMMARY

There is an urgent need to understand and optimize work–life integration for OMS. Progress in this area is likely to prevent individual burnout and attrition as well as retain a diverse workforce in OMS. Interventions at the individual, organizational and societal levels are critical to develop systemic changes.

CLINICS CARE POINTS

- Work–life integration is a worthwhile goal that can improve surgeon well-being, productivity, satisfaction, and patient outcomes.

- Burnout can manifest with physical or cognitive symptoms; signs of burnout include exhaustion, disengagement, hostility, cynicism, and depression.

- Individuals, societies, and organizations can implement strategies and programs that promote work–life balance; resources exist to assist in this goal such as the HBR Guide to Work–Life Balance[2] and the STEPS Forward Initiative.[45]

DISCLOSURE

The authors have nothing to disclose.

REFERENCES

1. Medscape national physician burnout & suicide report 2020: the generational divide. Available at: https://www.medscape.com/slideshow/2020-lifestyle-burnout-6012460. Accessed June 26, 2021.

2. Friedman F, Saunders E, Bergman P, et al. Harvard business review Guide to work life balance. Massachusetts: Harvard Business School Publishing Corporation; 2019.

3. Committee on systems approaches to improve patient care by supporting clinician well-being, National Academy of Medicine, National Academies of Sciences, Engineering, and Medicine. Taking action against clinician burnout: a systems approach to professional well-being. Washington, DC: National Academies Press; 2019. p. 2552.

4. Gander F, Proyer R, Ruch W. Positive psychology interventions addressing pleasure, engagement, meaning, positive relationships, and accomplishment increase well-being and ameliorate depressive symptoms: a randomized, placebo-controlled online study. Front Psychol 2016;7:686.

5. Smith C, Rao A, Tompach PC, et al. Factors associated with the mental health and satisfaction of oral and maxillofacial surgery residents in the united states: a cross-sectional study and analysis. J Oral Maxillofac Surg 2019;77(11):2196–204.

6. Lebares CC, Guvva EV, Ascher NL, et al. Burnout and stress among us surgery residents: psychological distress and resilience. J Am Coll Surg 2018; 226(1):80–90.

7. Kohnen J. Total leadership: be a better leader, have a richer life. Qual Manag J 2009;16(1):56.

8. Kent S, Herbert C, Magennis P, et al. What attracts people to a career in oral and maxillofacial surgery? A questionnaire survey. Br J Oral Maxillofac Surg 2017;55(1):41–5.

9. Stolarski A, Moseley JM, O'Neal P, et al. Retired surgeons' reflections on their careers. JAMA Surg 2020; 155(4):359.

10. Orri M, Farges O, Clavien P-A, et al. Being a surgeon—the myth and the reality: a meta-synthesis of surgeons' perspectives about factors affecting their practice and well-being. Ann Surg 2014; 260(5):721–9.

11. Bellodi PL. The general practitioner and the surgeon: stereotypes and medical specialties. Rev Hosp Clínicas 2004;59(1):15–24.

12. Chari R, Chang C-C, Sauter SL, et al. Expanding the paradigm of occupational safety and health: a new framework for worker well-being. J Occup Environ Med 2018;60(7):589–93.

13. Dyrbye LN, Freischlag J, Kaups KL, et al. Work-home conflicts have a substantial impact on career decisions that affect the adequacy of the surgical workforce. Arch Surg 2012;147(10):933–9.

14. Shapiro MC, Rao SR, Dean J, et al. Shame and burnout in oral and maxillofacial surgery resident education; a cross sectional analysis of 217 current OMS residents. J Oral Maxillofac Surg 2016;74(9): e38–9.

15. Maslach C, Jackson SE, Leiter MP. Maslach burnout inventory manual. Palo Alto, CA: Consulting Psychologists Press; 1996.

16. Shanafelt TD, Balch CM, Bechamps GJ, et al. Burnout and career satisfaction among American surgeons. Trans Meet Am Surg Assoc 2009;127:107–15.

17. Shanafelt TD, Dyrbye LN, Sinsky C, et al. Relationship between clerical burden and characteristics of the electronic environment with physician burnout and professional satisfaction. Mayo Clin Proc 2016; 91(7):836–48.

18. Shanafelt TD, Balch CM, Bechamps G, et al. Burnout and medical errors among American surgeons. Ann Surg 2010;251(6):995–1000.

19. Davis EC, Risucci DA, Blair PG, et al. Women in surgery residency programs: evolving trends from a national perspective. J Am Coll Surg 2011;212(3): 320–6.

20. Kolokythas A, Miloro M. Why do women choose to enter academic oral and maxillofacial surgery? J Oral Maxillofac Surg 2016;74(5):881–8.

21. Risser MJ, Laskin DM. Women in oral and maxillofacial surgery: factors affecting career choices, attitudes, and practice characteristics. J Oral Maxillofac Surg 1996;54(6):753–7.

22. Emslie C, Hunt K. 'Live to Work' or 'Work to Live'? A qualitative study of gender and work-life balance among men and women in mid-life. Gend Work Organ 2009;16(1):151–72.

23. Baptiste D, Fecher AM, Dolejs SC, et al. Gender differences in academic surgery, work-life balance, and satisfaction. J Surg Res 2017;218:99–107.

24. Dyrbye LN. Relationship between work-home conflicts and burnout among American surgeons: a comparison by sex. Arch Surg 2011;146(2):211.

25. Marti KC, Lanzon J, Edwards SP, et al. Career and professional satisfaction of oral and maxillofacial surgery residents, academic surgeons, and private practitioners: does gender matter? J Dent Educ 2017;81(1):75–86.

26. Sullivan MC, Yeo H, Roman SA, et al. Striving for work-life balance: effect of marriage and children on the experience of 4402 US general surgery residents. Ann Surg 2013;257(3):571–6.

27. Heisler CA, Miller P, Stephens EH, et al. Leading from behind: paucity of gender equity statements and policies among professional surgical societies. Am J Surg 2020;220(5):1132–5.

28. Mayer KL, Ho HS, Goodnight JE. Childbearing and child care in surgery. Arch Surg 2001;136(6): 649–55.

29. Osseo-Asare A, Balasuriya L, Huot SJ, et al. Minority resident physicians' views on the role of race/ethnicity in their training experiences in the workplace. JAMA Netw Open 2018;1(5):e182723.

30. Peterson NB, Friedman RH, Ash AS, et al. Faculty self-reported experience with racial and ethnic discrimination in academic medicine. J Gen Intern Med 2004;19(3):259–65.

31. Garcia LC, Shanafelt TD, West CP, et al. Burnout, depression, career satisfaction, and work-life integration by physician race/ethnicity. JAMA Netw Open 2020;3(8):e2012762.

32. Dyrbye LN, Burke SE, Hardeman RR, et al. Association of clinical specialty with symptoms of burnout and career choice regret among US resident physicians. JAMA 2018;320(11):1114.

33. Afzal KI, Khan FM, Mulla Z, et al. Primary language and cultural background as factors in resident burnout in medical specialties: a study in a bilingual US city. South Med J 2010;103(7):607–15.

34. Meredith LS, Schmidt Hackbarth N, Darling J, et al. Emotional exhaustion in primary care during early implementation of the VA's medical home transformation: patient-aligned care team (PACT). Med Care 2015;53(3):253–60.

35. Dyrbye LN, Thomas MR, Eacker A, et al. Race, ethnicity, and medical student well-being in the United States. Arch Intern Med 2007;167(19):2103.

36. Aziz SR. Racial diversity in American oral and maxillofacial surgery. J Oral Maxillofac Surg 2010;68(8): 1723–31.

37. Criddle T-R, Gordon NC, Blakey G, et al. African Americans in oral and maxillofacial surgery: factors affecting career choice, satisfaction, and practice patterns. J Oral Maxillofac Surg 2017;75(12): 2489–96.

38. Eisemann B, Wagner R, Reece E. Practical negotiation for medical professionals. Semin Plast Surg 2018;32(04):166–71.

39. Guetter CR, McGuire KP, Oropallo AR, et al. Surgical job negotiations: how current literature and expert opinion can inform your strategies. Am J Surg 2020;220(5):1201–7.

40. West CP, Dyrbye LN, Sinsky C, et al. Resilience and burnout among physicians and the general US working population. JAMA Netw Open 2020;3(7): e209385.

41. Lebares CC, Hershberger AO, Guvva EV, et al. Feasibility of formal mindfulness-based stress-resilience training among surgery interns: a randomized clinical trial. JAMA Surg 2018;153(10):e182734.

42. Shanafelt TD, Kaups KL, Nelson H, et al. An interactive individualized intervention to promote behavioral change to increase personal well-being in US surgeons. Ann Surg 2014;259(1):82–8.

43. West CP, Dyrbye LN, Erwin PJ, et al. Interventions to prevent and reduce physician burnout: a systematic review and meta-analysis. The Lancet 2016; 388(10057):2272–81.

44. Panagioti M, Panagopoulou E, Bower P, et al. Controlled interventions to reduce burnout in physicians: a systematic review and meta-analysis. JAMA Intern Med 2017;177(2):195.

45. AMA steps forward. Available at: Https://Edhub. Ama-Assn.Org/Steps-Forward. Accessed January 27, 2021.

46. National Academies of Sciences, Engineering, and Medicine. Taking action against clinician burnout: a systems approach to professional well-being. Washington, DC: The National Academies Press; 2019.

47. Kemp MT, Rivard SJ, Anderson S, et al. Trainee wellness and safety in the context of COVID-19: the experience of one institution. Acad Med 2020; 96(5):655–60.

48. Shanafelt TD, Gorringe G, Menaker R, et al. Impact of organizational leadership on physician burnout and satisfaction. Mayo Clin Proc 2015;90(4):432–40.

49. Altieri MS, Salles A, Bevilacqua LA, et al. Perceptions of surgery residents about parental leave during training. JAMA Surg 2019;154(10):952.

Effects of the COVID-19 Pandemic on the Professional Career of Women in Oral and Maxillofacial Surgery

Rachel Bishop, DDS, MD[a], Jennifer E. Woerner, DMD, MD[a], Franci Stavropoulos, DDS[b],*

KEYWORDS

- COVID-19 pandemic • Women in oral and maxillofacial surgery (OMS) • Implicit bias • Pay disparity
- Gender inequity • Physician burnout • Virtual education format

KEY POINTS

- The devastating effects of the COVID-19 pandemic have affected people worldwide. Women in the workforce have been inordinately impacted by the pandemic. Female oral and maxillofacial surgeons (OMS) faced evident barriers and biases before the pandemic that are now exacerbated. The COVID-19 pandemic has revealed these disparities.
- Quarantine and stay-at-home orders played a significant role in the hardships that women OMS face because of increased burden of domestic and childcare obligations.
- Established salary inequality for women physicians becomes more evident during a pandemic and ultimately impacts the potential academic promotion and financial success of women OMS.
- The COVID-19 pandemic has worsened burnout globally, and women physicians are disproportionately bearing the burden.
- Lack of in-person symposiums, interviews, and externship opportunities limits the potential for women to intermingle, provide mentorship, and foster an environment for equality.
- the preexisting inequities within the OMS specialty and the likely exacerbation of these inequities by the COVID-19 pandemic, there is an invitation for OMS programs across the United States to provide transparency during policy implementation and incorporate women into leadership positions whereby policies are created that ultimately influence future lives and careers of women in OMS.

THE COVID-19 PANDEMIC

Coronavirus disease 2019 (COVID-19 is the infection that results from contracting the novel coronavirus (severe acute respiratory syndrome coronavirus 2 or SARS-CoV-2).[1] As of June 2021, 169 million people worldwide have contracted the virus, and there have been a staggering 3.5 million deaths.[2] COVID-19 has become the third leading cause of death in the United States, following heart disease and cancer. The lives of individuals around the world were altered by the devastating effects of the COVID-19 pandemic. To aid in reducing transmission of the coronavirus, nonessential workers were quarantined, followed by stay-at-home orders and travel restrictions

a Department of Oral and Maxillofacial Surgery, Louisiana State University Health Sciences Center-Shreveport, 1501 Kings Highway, Room 503, Shreveport, LA 71103, USA; b Department of Oral & Maxillofacial Surgery, Oregon Health & Science University, School of Dentistry, 2730 SW Moody Avenue, Portland, OR 97201, USA
* Corresponding author.
E-mail address: stavropo@ohsu.edu

Oral Maxillofacial Surg Clin N Am 33 (2021) 475–480
https://doi.org/10.1016/j.coms.2021.06.002
1042-3699/21/© 2021 Elsevier Inc. All rights reserved.

flourished.[3] Health care professionals were considered "essential" workers, and stay-at-home orders excluded them. Lack of personal protective equipment (PPE), exposure to the coronavirus, and risk of infection altered life on a fundamental level.

Many of the US workforce have at least 1 child, and many without institutional childcare were forced to leave the workforce to provide for children at home.[4] As a result, the coronavirus uniquely affected the female workforce and, in particular, women in medicine. A prevention article published in "Innovations and Provocations" highlights that the reproductive age of women overlaps with their early academic careers, expanding the loss of women through the "academic pipeline."[5] This finding was also noted in an opinion piece by D. M. Laskin published in 2015 wherein Laskin stated that the "desire of women to eventually raise a family" often precludes them from the academic setting and funnels women into the private practice sector.[6] The barriers for women and the scarcity of instrumental policies that should be created to support women in academic medicine who also have children must be considered, as many women during the pandemic have been forced to carry the burden of domiciliary obligations. These factors are an essential consideration when studying the effects of the pandemic on female medical professionals.

The COVID-19 pandemic has affected physicians across the globe, specifically oral and maxillofacial surgeons (OMS). Surgeries involving the head and neck region increase the risk of virus transmission. This worldwide health crisis shifted the health care system's priorities from treatment of all medical ailments to only emergent and urgent conditions. This transformation affected both attending physicians and residents. In a survey published in the *Journal of Oral and Maxillofacial Surgery*, it was found that OMS residents were concerned about meeting graduation requirements because of canceled elective cases and programs that shifted to virtual-only education, and residents had limited access to adequate PPE resources, including N95 respirators.[7] PPE and respirators are known to have specific fit issues for the female gender, further increasing the risk of contracting coronavirus for women surgeons. The above concerns combined with women comprising a greater majority of junior clinical appointments compared with men increases exposure of women to COVID-19.[8] OMS conferences across the United States were canceled, and virtual symposiums became the norm. Although the virtual platform could increase global educational opportunities for many,[9] special interest groups suffered, specifically those geared toward women, such as the women's special interest group at the American Association of Oral and Maxillofacial Surgeons (AAOMS) annual meeting. In addition, an article submitted to "Academic Medicine" discussed gender equity issues stating that women may be spoken over in virtual formats and even interrupted more often. The lack of in person events and its consequences stifle professional opportunities and recognition for minorities such as women.[10] Furthermore, virtual formats for symposiums limit the informal networking opportunities that could previously be expected. These factors coupled with the unique roles that women play in both academia and home life resulted in the coronavirus having a disproportionate impact on women.

GENDER INEQUITY IN THE SPECIALTY

Gender imbalance is common among most surgical specialties in the United States, with women comprising only a small minority of the surgical workforce.[11] The paucity of active women in OMS participating at the national level is evident, with female participants of AAOMS and American College of Oral and Maxillofacial Surgeons being only 8% and 10%, respectively.[12] In order to analyze the reasons for the scarceness of women in oral surgery and its impact, one must consider the process of becoming an oral surgeon, starting with dental school. Many sacrifices must be made in order to gain acceptance to an oral surgery program. Matriculation necessitates decreased family time, increased hours dedicated to the oral surgery service at one's dental school and thus preparing for the comprehensive basic sciences examination (which is the standard metric used to distinguish candidates), and increased hours participating in several externships. All of these factors are required to exhibit true dedication and preparedness. In a survey conducted on the perception of women in the field, Rostami and Laskin[13] noted that a potential reason for the disparity of women in OMS could be attributed to a low applicant pool as opposed to implicit bias among program directors at OMS programs. However, Rostami and Laskin also found that male residents did have biases against their female counterparts, and they were concerned that the reason for the difference in responses among residents and program directors could be because of leaders in the specialty answering with only "socially acceptable viewpoints rather than the true condition." Quandary begs the question, what then are the underlying difficulties that influence women to forego applying to an OMS program?

Gender bias starts early in the career of a female OMS, as early as dental school. As Rostami and Laskin stated: "Although most practicing surgeons, residents, and program directors agreed that women are as capable as men to practice OMS, there continues to be some bias against women in the field." This analysis by Rostami and Laskin included the conclusion by Brunner and Campbell, that this bias was also a perception of female dental students.[13] A survey published in the *Journal of Oral and Maxillofacial Surgery* in 2019 focusing on the sexual harassment of women concluded that sexually harassing behavior of women is prevalent, and it "erodes [their] personal confidence and career development."[14] This award-winning abstract was also the subject of a 2019 editorial published in *Forbes* and submitted to the Academic Surgical Congress by a team from the University of North Carolina. The survey regarded the harassment and bullying of female surgeons. It was revealed that 58% of women surgeons, in the year leading up to the survey, experienced sexual harassment. Interestingly, "the majority (84%) of incidents of harassment reported by women as part of the survey were not reported to any institutional authority." The reason? Fear. "Fear of negative impact on career (43%), fear of retribution (32%), and fear of being dismissed and/or inaction towards the perpetrator (31%)."[15,16] The problem is 2-fold: women are experiencing harassment, which can affect all aspects of one's surgical production and success, and women feel they cannot report these issues without inflicting increased damage on their already precarious careers. This issue is a social issue, at best, and a safety issue at worst. It is imperative to analyze findings such as these, as historical norms and trends only become more evident and prevalent in times of crisis, such as the COVID-19 pandemic. Examination must be made of how women fared before the pandemic to understand the subsequent inequities that surface and escalate afterward.

Women are often encouraged to pursue career paths other than surgery. Despite women making up 50% or greater of the populace of US dental schools, there is still a disproportionate number of women who choose not to pursue surgical residency.[17] Women who enter surgical residency forego careers in academic medicine. Attributed reasons for this could be the lack of leadership roles available to women, decreased pay for equal effort, and the preexisting biases regarding motherhood. An Ontario study also reported that women in surgery are paid 24% less per hour than their male counterparts.[18] In the United States, women physicians earn 75 cents on the dollar compared with men. This pay disparity is one of the largest in any profession.[19] Disparity in earnings and the lack of leadership roles for women are just 2 of the many factors influencing women to forego academic surgical careers. In 2018, Debra M. Sajcco, DMD, MD was the first woman elected to the AAOMS Board of Trustees, despite AAOMS originating in the year 1918,[20] which indicates the impediment of the male-dominated OMS field to diversify leadership.

QUARANTINE ISSUES FOR WOMEN IN ORAL AND MAXILLOFACIAL SURGERY

Pandemic quarantine issues were vastly different for women than their male counterparts. Women typically assume a greater amount of the domestic duties at home and care for children and elderly on average more than men.[8] This increased burden alone decreases the time that women are attributing to their career and academic aspirations. During the COVID-19 pandemic, this issue is compounded by the fact that daycares and schools were closed. Many female academicians were sequestered to home, quarantined with children who required attention and care, further decreasing a woman's academic productivity. Although COVID-19 affected men also, women were in the majority of those assuming traditional duties at home. School closings and self-isolation at home necessitated women sacrificing their academic work for responsibilities in the household.[10] Unpaid childcare is often devalued and exploited, which further pervades the gender pay disparity[21]; this permeates all areas of advancement for women when combined with inherent biases in the work place.

PAY GAP AND TENURE TRACK

The concerns encompassing the gender pay gap must be assessed by considering all factors that contribute to delays in academic progression. The family household and childcare burdens of women diminish the time and effort women are able to contribute to their career. Placing the onus on women influences the time allocated to writing research papers and applying for grants, which directly affects achieving tenure and potential career advancement. Although women increased their contributions to coauthored research before the pandemic, their presence as first author has continued to dwindle. Article submissions during COVID-19 have shown a decreased female presence, and this includes both coauthorship and first-author positions.[4] The lack of authorship affects a female surgeon's ability to climb the tenure ladder and alters potential raises in salary. Subsequently, women have less resources for retirement and investments. In addition to women contributing to fewer publications and having less time for authorship, women are overlooked for their service and committee participant contributions. All of these factors combined decreases and delays potential tenure achievement, as research, teaching, and clinical time are regarded with more esteem.[5] Women are more often involved in unpaid committees and service opportunities that progress the specialty, yet these contributions are not weighted as heavily as research contributions, further widening both the promotion and the pay gap.[5,19,22]

In an editorial regarding gender wage gap, it was noted that "because women tend to work fewer hours to accommodate caregiving and other unpaid obligations, they are also more likely to work part-time, which means lower hourly wages and fewer benefits compared with full-time workers."[23] Tenure leads to increased pay, promotional opportunities, and academic freedom. When women are not afforded these opportunities, it limits the advancement of women in the specialty. These key issues culminate in women becoming sole caretakers, missing more work, logging less hours at work, qualifying for less benefits, and being offered fewer promotions and prospects. According to an article written in *Sustainability: Science, Practice and Policy*, "Women are also less likely to have a financial safety net, due to greater job insecurity and lower average pay rates for women."[21] Interestingly, a *New York Times* editorial published in 2020 embellishing on the research findings that women undergo harsher end of contract evaluations concluded "women and people of color are more likely than men to get comments related to their appearance or the tone of their voice," factors that have no relation to one's ability to teach. It was also noted that these unjust criticisms could intensify during the pandemic.[22] Women are trapped in an inescapable gender-bias whirlpool culminating in the loss of career advancement and financial success, resulting in their male counterparts flourishing and women floundering.

Women who contribute more time to clinical and surgical education and who focus on committee work are particularly disadvantaged, as these activities are not weighted as heavily as research and grant approvals for the traditional tenure track. During the pandemic, women who were able to continue surgical duties continued to be exposed to coronavirus at an increased rate than their male colleagues. Some physicians saw a clear gender disparity in patients being treated for post-COVID-19 conditions as "long haulers,"

with women facing higher rates of chronic conditions.[24] The potential increase in viral exposure combined with the chronicity of illness could result in decreased time at work contributing to surgical and clinical teaching and decreased attention to academic research thus limiting the chances of progression.

PHYSICIAN BURNOUT

The COVID-19 pandemic increased the already high incidence of physician burnout among women. Although the pandemic contributed to physician burnout across both genders, women were disproportionally affected.[8] According to a descriptive study recently published in *JAMA Network*, "women surgeons experience less achievement, are more dissatisfied, and have higher levels of burnout compared with their male colleagues."[25] Burnout decreases production, increases errors at work, and decreases motivation. If burnout is affecting women at a greater incidence than men, it is axiomatic that women will suffer greater consequences in the academic and surgical arena. Anecdotally but also supported by the findings of Rostami and Laskin,[13] women are perceived as weaker and less emotionally stable than men. These fallacies can result in "imposter syndrome" and the quest to stay one step ahead of their male counterparts to be viewed as "at par," fostering additional burnout. A survey published in *The Journal of Surgical Education* highlights this concept, finding that women "trainees in male dominate specialties were more likely to report gender bias …may leave medicine/retire early, and would not recommend [the] profession to trainees or family members."[26] The prejudice experienced by women is a compounding and unfortunate issue, as less women in OMS will recommend the specialty to their colleagues, further exacerbating the gender discrepancy. These matters are only amplified during a pandemic where both genders experience additional burnout and fatigue.

LACK OF IN-PERSON MEETINGS, INTERVIEWS, EXTERNSHIPS

Recently, women have organized to form special interest groups, such as the women's special interest group at AAOMS. Due to COVID-19, the special interest group was completely removed from the virtual forum AAOMS used for their 2020 annual meeting. COVID-19 continues to decrease past progression of women in the specialty. With fewer opportunities for women to comingle with like-minded individuals for support and advice, women are left without significant mentors and role models. Lacking female leadership and attendings in OMS only perpetuates pre-existing biases. The overall lack of female promotion results in less women in leadership roles where influential and consequential decisions are made.[27] Ultimately, the deficiency of women in leadership positions at universities and medical centers distances women from discussions regarding important policies, such as maternity leave, paid leave, childcare options, and other benefits that specifically affect women. COVID-19 will further exacerbate these matters, as there will be decreased funding for grants and potential departmental funds. Women will be the first on the chopping block.

The inability for women to be physically present at externships, interviews, and symposiums decreases chances for acceptance. When women are afforded the opportunity to interact with their male counterparts, they are able to exhibit their proficiency, knowledge, and expertise in their field. Female representation, in turn, results in greater reception of women in the surgical workforce and debunks myths regarding women and their ability to perform as well as men.

SUMMARY

The COVID-19 pandemic did not create the gender disparity in pay, opportunity, and academic advancement, but it has exacerbated it and highlighted those areas where the inequity exists. In order to combat the issues encompassing implicit bias that cultivates an environment where women struggle to excel, education must be rendered to ensure that those in the profession are cognizant that these inequities do exist. Childcare at work and paid leave to care for children at home are just some of the many options that must be made available to women. Tenure tracks must include all academic roles, including service and committee work as ways to ascend the tenure path. Extension of the tenure timeline must also be considered. Women need a seat at the table when influential decisions are being made and policies are implemented. These policies ultimately affect women's ability to adequately have work-life balance with continued path for progress and success. Transparency is key, and women OMS should have a voice in the decision-making processes, especially when establishing criteria for salary promotion and tenure achievement. Women should have the opportunity to serve in leadership positions, both for mentorship of female surgeons to come and to aid in making decisions that affect all surgeons. Women can help facilitate the difficult

discussions and assist in resolving implicit gender bias. Until the time comes when "female" is not a prefix to "surgeon," gender inequity will not be overcome. Rostami and colleagues[17] wrote that there has been an increased representation of women in both residency training programs and practice, but highlighted the ever-present bias, sexual harassment, and social dilemmas that discourage women from choosing OMS as a specialty. Although women have progressed since the early days of Elaine Steubner's tenure (the first female OMS, graduating residency in 1958), the specialty and women still have a long way to go.

DISCLOSURE STATEMENT

The authors have no conflicts of interest, disclosures, or financial interests in any matter or material discussed in the article.

REFERENCES

1. World Health Organization. Transmission of SARS-CoV-2: implications for infection prevention precautions: scientific brief. Geneva: World Health Organization; 2020. Available at: https://www.who.int/newsroom/commentaries/detail/transmission-of-sars-cov-2-implications-for-infection-prevention-precautions. Accessed May 28, 2021.
2. The worldometer. Available at: https://www.worldometers.info/coronavirus/coronavirus-death-toll/. Accessed May 28, 2021.
3. Gostin LO, Chertoff MJ. Lockdowns, quarantines, and travel restrictions, during COVID and beyond: what's the law, and how should we decide? Health Aff Blog 2021. Available at: https://www.health affairs.org/do/10.1377/hblog20210322.450239/full/. Accessed May 27, 2021.
4. Krukowski RA, Jagsi R, Cardel MI. Academic productivity differences by gender and child age in science, technology, engineering, mathematics, and medicine faculty during the COVID-19 pandemic. J Womens Health 2020;30(3):341–7.
5. Cardel MI, Dean N, Montoya-Williams D. Preventing a secondary epidemic of lost early career scientists. Effects of COVID-19 pandemic on women with children. Ann Am Thorac Soc 2020;17(11):1366–70.
6. Laskin DM. The role of women in academic oral and maxillofacial surgery. J Oral Maxillofac Surg 2015;73(4):579.
7. Huntley RE, Ludwig DC, Dillon JK. Early effects of COVID-19 on oral and maxillofacial surgery residency training—results from a national survey. J Oral Maxillofac Surg 2020;78(8):1257–67.
8. Madsen TE, Dobiesz V, Das D, et al. Unique risks and solutions for equitable advancement during the Covid-19 pandemic: early experience from

frontline physicians in academic medicine. NEJM Catalyst Innov Care Deliv 2020;1(4).

9. Maffia F, Fesenko II, Vellone V. Covid-2019 pandemic: growing wave of cancelled meetings in oral and maxillofacial surgery and its impact on specialty. J Diagn Treat Oral Maxillofacial Pathol 2020. https://doi.org/10.23999/j.dtomp.2020.7.1.

10. Woitowich NC, Jain S, Arora VM, et al. COVID-19 threatens progress toward gender equity within academic medicine. Acad Med J Assoc Am Med Colleges 2021;96(6):813–6.

11. Aziz HL, Ducoin C, Welsh D, et al. 2018 ACS Governors Survey: gender inequality and harassment remain a challenge in surgery. Chicago: The American College of Surgeons Bulletin Brief; 2019. Available at: https://bulletin.facs.org/2019/09/2018-acs-governors-survey-gender-inequality-and-harassment-remain-a-challenge-in-surgery/.

12. Drew SJ. Women as oral and maxillofacial surgeons: past, present, and future. In: President's editorial—American College of Oral and Maxillofacial Surgeons (ACOMS). 2018. Available at: https://www.acoms.org/news/407850/Presidents-Editorial.htm 2018. Accessed May 27, 2021.

13. Rostami F, Laskin DM. Male perception of women in oral and maxillofacial surgery. J Oral Maxillofac Surg 2014;72(12):2383–5.

14. Zurayk LF, Cheng KL, Zemplenyi M, et al. Perceptions of sexual harassment in oral and maxillofacial surgery training and practice. J Oral Maxillofac Surg 2019;77(12):2377–85.

15. Lee BY. 58% of women surgeons suffer sexual harassment: why this may hurt you too. Jersey City: Forbes; 2019. Available at: https://www.forbes.com/sites/brucelee/2019/02/16/why-58-of-women-surgeons-experiencing-sexual-harassment-may-hurt-you/. Accessed May 30, 2021.

16. Nayyar A, Scarlet S, Strassle PD, et al. A national survey of sexual harassment among surgeons. In: 14th annual academic surgical congress, Houston, Texas. 2019.

17. Rostami F, Ahmed AE, Best AM, et al. The changing personal and professional characteristics of women in oral and maxillofacial surgery. J Oral Maxillofac Surg 2010;68(2):381–5.

18. Dossa F, Simpson AN, Sutradhar R, et al. Sex-based disparities in the hourly earnings of surgeons in the fee-for-service system in Ontario, Canada. JAMA Surg 2019;154(12):1134–42.

19. Narayana S, Roy B, Merriam S, et al. Minding the gap: organizational strategies to promote gender equity in academic medicine during the COVID-19 pandemic. J Gen Intern Med 2020;35(12):3681–4.

20. Lew D. A historical overview of the AAOMS. Rosemont, (IL): American Association of Oral and Maxillofacial Surgeons; 2013. Available at: https://www.aaoms.org/images/uploads/pdfs/historical_overview_aaoms.pdf.

21. Power K. The COVID-19 pandemic has increased the care burden of women and families. Sustainability 2020;16(1):67–73.

22. Kramer J. The virus moved female faculty to the Brink. Will universities help? New York: The New York Times; 2020. Available at: https://www.nytimes.com/2020/10/06/science/covid-universities-women.html. Accessed May 27, 2021.

23. Bleiweis R. Quick facts about the gender wage gap. Washington, DC: Center for American Progress; 2020. Available at: https://www.americanprogress.org/issues/women/reports/2020/03/24/482141/quick-facts-gender-wage-gap/. Accessed May 27, 2021.

24. Youn S. Way more women are reporting 'long-haul' covid symptoms. In: Doctors aren't sure why. The Lilly; 2021. Available at: https://www.thelily.com/way-more-women-are-reporting-long-haul-covid-symptoms-doctors-arent-sure-why/. Accessed May 28, 2021.

25. Dossett LA, Vitous CA, Lindquist K, et al. Women surgeons' experiences of interprofessional workplace conflict. JAMA Netw Open 2020;3(10):e2019843.

26. Barnes KL, McGuire L, Dunivan G, et al. Gender bias experiences of female surgical trainees. J Surg Educ 2019;76(6):e1–14.

27. Jones Y, Durand V, Moron K, et al. Collateral damage: how COVID-19 is adversely impacting women physicians. J Hosp Med 2020;15(8):507–9.

Where Are the Women
Evolution of Women's Specialty Organizations

Jane A. Petro, MD*

KEYWORDS

- Women in surgical subspecialties • Entering the workforce • History of women who were firsts

KEY POINTS

- Women in the nineteenth century fought to create a space within the medical and dental profession.
- The first 50 years, seeing a gradual increase in both numbers and acceptance was followed by a sharp decline in both.
- After the Civil Rights Act of 1964, women again began to find space in the profession.
- The 1980s saw the emergence of women-specific subspecialty organizations creating space for female participation.
- A more robust effort for diversity, inclusion, and equality has followed the TIME'S UP Healthcare Movement after 2015.

INTRODUCTION

In the mid-nineteenth century small numbers of women began entering the professions. These numbers increased slowly but steadily through the beginning of the twentieth century, only to decline with the advent of coeducation and the closing of women-only programs and institutions. Dentistry never formed women's dental schools, with coeducational schools available in small numbers after the 1870s. National women's professional associations began forming with the American Medical Women's Association (AMWA) in 1915 and the Federation of Women Dentists in 1921. (In 1892, the Women's Dental Association was formed with 12 members. This organization grew to more than 100 members, but ceased to exist for unknown reasons in 1898.) AMWA formed from an amalgam of local women physicians groups, to address and document unequal opportunities for women physicians. The Federation of Women Dentists (FWD) formed in 1921 under the direction of Vida Latham, DDS, MD, the year following her admission to the American Dental Association. The FWD (now the American Association of Women Dentists) had as its stated goal to form a support organization to share common interests, friendship, and camaraderie. The FWD evolved, becoming an advocacy organization after World War II when many women dentists were displaced by returning veterans. In this article, the evolution of women's participation within the surgical subspecialties will be examined, including both the medical and dental organizations.

There was a gradual decline in women entering the professions during the first 60 years of the twentieth century, followed by a relatively robust increase. In 1900, nearly 70 of 1000 physicians were women, but by 1920, it had declined to 50 of 1000.[1] In 1905, 4% of all medical school graduates were women, but by 1915, this had decreased to 2.6%; 9% of medical students were women by 1969. In dental education, women's representation remained low, with women representing 0.9% of first year dental students in 1968 to 1969.[2]

What changed in the 1960s and the 1970s that resulted in increasing women's admission to medical and dental education? Most writers agree that

Emerita New York Medical College, Valhalla, NY, USA
* 40 A Pond Street, Jamaica Plain, MA 02130.
E-mail address: drjpetro@aol.com

Oral Maxillofacial Surg Clin N Am 33 (2021) 481–489
https://doi.org/10.1016/j.coms.2021.05.007
1042-3699/21/© 2021 Elsevier Inc. All rights reserved.

the emergence of feminism in the 1960s, along with the publication of "The Feminine Mystique" in 1963, changed the conversation about women's roles in the home, and in society. Campbell and McCammon[1] contend that by 1910, medical schools with their limited quotas for women and cultural norms discouraged women from participation in rigorous careers. These quotas were "potent barriers to women's pursuit of medicine as a vocation." If cultural barriers were also significant, then necessary changes in cultural norms appeared in the 1970s with the emerging civil rights movement.

President John F. Kennedy initiated the nationwide conversation about civil rights in his June 11, 1963, speech to the nation, after months of civil unrest. In addressing civil rights issues, Kennedy framed equal opportunity as a moral issue. And although Kennedy primarily was addressing African American civil rights, the civil rights legislation, when it was passed a year later, not only ended segregation in public places but also banned discrimination on the basis of race, color, religion, sex, or national origin. Signed into law by Lyndon Johnson on July 2, 1964, the Civil Rights Act, by banning gender discrimination, opened the door for women to demand access. This accidental inclusion of gender equality in an amendment to the Act was offered in an attempt to defeat the law but ended up being included when the law was passed an hour later.[3]

WOMEN SURGEONS/WOMEN ORAL SURGEONS

Twentieth century arguments about the dangers of admitting women to the profession, especially surgery, were often based on child bearing. In 1975, James Haug, an executive in the American College of Surgeons (ACS), stated, "The interruptions in a woman's medical career due to marriage or maternity have raised questions concerning the cost effectiveness of their medical training."[4] In telling the stories of women surgeons in the United States, "gender discrimination," "widespread bias against women training in surgery," and "absence of role models and mentors" describe their common experiences.[5]

Are prevailing attitudes against women part of the reason they have entered the surgical profession so slowly? Reasons offered for these disparities include gendered expectations about work/life balance, long residencies with inflexible scheduling, and lack of parental leave policies. Fitzgerald and colleagues[6] screened for the presence of sexual harassment, abuse, and discrimination within surgical residencies in 2019. This study found that 28.9% of respondents (91% female) experienced sexual harassment, primarily from senior male supervising physicians with only a quarter of these incidents being reported.[6] The investigators concluded, "Work is needed to not only change the common perception that abuse is a normal part of surgical training….research would be needed to examine the impact of discrimination and harassment on resident attrition and medical student interest in surgery as a career choice."

Work life balance is frequently cited as a significant deterrent to women's professional success. Many of the twentieth century pioneers in surgery and oral surgery were unmarried and childless as the following brief descriptions of "First Women" show.

Mary Edwards Walker, MD (1832–1919): The only woman to serve as a surgeon in the Civil War and the only woman to be awarded the Congressional Medal of Honor, the United States' highest military award.

Bertha van Hoosen, MD (1863–1952): Founding president of AMWA, first woman to be head of a surgical department in a coeducational medical school as Professor and Chair of Gynecology at Loyola University in 1918.

Lilliam Ketrua Pond Farrar, MD (1871–1962): First woman Fellow of the American Gynecologic Society, first woman to serve as Governor of the American College of Surgeons (1925–1938), founding Diplomat of the American Board of Obstetrics & Gynecology.

Olga Jonasson, MD (1934–2006): First woman to hold a high-level staff position with the American College of Surgeons in 1993; first woman to head the surgical section of a major city hospital, Cook County in 1977; first woman to chair an academic surgery department at Ohio State University 1987 to 1993.

Alma Dea Morani, MD (1907–2001): First woman admitted to the American Society Plastic and Reconstructive Surgery (ASPRS, later ASPS), clinical professor of surgery and plastic surgery at Women's Medical College of Pennsylvania in 1948, and founded the first hand surgery specialty clinic in Pennsylvania.

Ruth Jackson, MD (1902–1994): First woman to complete an orthopedic residency in 1932, first to be board certified in 1937, and first to be admitted to the American Academy of Orthopedic Surgeons (AAOS) in 1937.

Louise Eisenhardt, MD (1891–1969): A neuropathologist and close collaborator with Harvey Cushing, MD, and the first woman to be president of the American Association of Neurological Surgeons (AANS) in 1938.

Vida Latham, MD, DDS (1866–1958): Pioneer whose research on oral tumors, surgery, and anatomy and whose role as author and journal editor actively promoted women in both dentistry and medicine. She was one of the founders of the Federation of Women Dentists that became the American Association of Woman Dentists.

Elaine Alice Stuebner, DDS (1908–2007): First woman member of the AAOMS, first woman to graduate in oral and maxillofacial surgery (OMS) from Cook County Hospital in 1958, first to be certified by the American Board of Oral and Maxillofacial Surgery (ABOMS), and in 1960, the first woman to join the American College of Oral Maxillofacial Surgery (ACOMS). Stuebner was a renowned clinician, a mentor, an academic, and author. It was 25 years before another woman entered the field of OMS.[7]

Nina Braunwald, MD (1928–1992): First female general surgeon at Bellvue, first woman cardiovascular surgeon, first woman certified by the American Board of Thoracic Surgery, and first person to develop and implant a mitral valve. She is the only woman among these giants whose firsts were accomplished while being married and raising 3 daughters.

As women moved in larger numbers into the medical profession, changes in representation among specialties also emerged with clear gendered distinctions between male and female fields of practice. A similar pattern had emerged in the early 1900s. Martha Tracy, MD (1876–1942) surveyed women physicians in 1921 and found a high percentage of them were entering specialties, primarily those related directly to women and children, or in public health, which she characterized as specific to women's interests.[8] These trends continue to be seen with significant disproportion between male and female specialty choices in the twenty-first century. Women represent 45.6% of graduate medical education (GME) trainees in the United States (2019 data), whereas they are disproportionately low among the specialties. In comparing the gender gap within 20 Accreditation Council for Graduate Medical Education (ACGME)-accredited specialties, otolaryngology, plastic surgery, urology, orthopedic, and neurosurgery had the lowest quartile of representation. In contrast, obstetrics and gynecology with 82% women, pediatrics with 70% women, dermatology with 64% women, and internal medicine, family medicine, and psychiatry each with 54% women contrast sharply with all the surgical fields.[9]

Pioneers in dental surgery emerged later in the twentieth century reflecting their lower participation in dental school, and significant disproportion

continues to exist. In 2004, 19% of practicing dentists were women, whereas a decade later, this increased to 29.8%. By 2018, 50% of dental DDS students were women. Gender diversification after completion of training indicates that women in dentistry are still more likely than men to treat primarily women and children and to provide services to underserved patient communities.[10] In addition, the wage gap for women remains significantly large.[11] The gender gap is the greatest among OMF surgeons. As of 2015, 12% of OMS residents were women and only 6% of AAOMS members were women. This figure compares to 67% of oral medicine residents and 62% of pediatric dentistry residents who are female.[12] As Natalie Eden notes, now women represent 31% of practicing dentists, but only 8% of AAOMS members and 10% of ACOMS members.[13] In contrast, 20% of general surgeons are women, whereas 40% of general surgical residents are women.[14]

As women's participation in professional organizations in the 1970s and the 1980s increased, many women saw a need for unique women's sections with or separate from their specialty organization. In a review of the role such women's groups could play, Kohman and Hoefer[15] examined 9 women's specialty groups that represented a female membership, which had never had an organizational voice, served in any elective offices, and often not even on or as committee chairs within their specialty. The investigators observed a common theme among these groups: an origin from a casual meeting held during their national specialty society annual meeting and later formalizing, with by-laws, and elected officials.[15] Among these groups, including orthopedics, cardiothoracic surgery, and oral maxillofacial surgery, it was nearly 25 years from the entry of the first woman into the specialty society until another woman joined.

ASSOCIATION OF WOMEN SURGEONS

The first contemporary surgical association for women began in 1981 and became the Association of Women Surgeons (AWS). A casual breakfast meeting was organized by Patricia Numann, MD FACS. Dr Numann has numerous "firsts" in surgery, including the first woman to receive the ACS Distinguished Service Award in 2006. After being denied surgical residency by many programs, Dr Numann was accepted by a program, initiating an exceptional career as an endocrine surgeon and full professor.[16]

In founding the AWS, Dr Numann invited as many women surgeons as she could identify to a breakfast meeting during the annual American College of Surgeons meeting. These meetings represented *"the first significant contact that many female residents or newly practicing female surgeons has with more professionally advance surgical women was through these Wednesday morning breakfasts at the ACS fall meeting"* according to Dr Numann. As AWS grew, the need for a specific separate identity led to incorporation in 1986, and a membership drive brought the group to nearly 1000 members 2 years later. Despite this progress, 96% of women surgeons surveyed in 1990 still considered surgery as unfavorable toward their gender, as opposed to 0% of men.[17] The AWS has grown to more than 3000 members with programs that include research scholarships, traveling visiting professorships, and gender-specific residency evaluations.[18] The benefits of these programs have been shown in several ways. The research grants given out between 1996 and 2020 to 24 individuals totaled $596,700. Subsequent NIH funding to those individuals reached $6,611,927, a return on investment resulting in significant numbers of publications and high index and impact factor ratings.[19] Women have entered the leadership of the American College of Surgeons, with 22 Department Chairs, members of the Board of Governors of the ACS, and 3 have become presidents of the ACS. The AWS has played a significant role in promoting women within the ACS, in increasing the number of women in residency programs, and in discussions of salary equity, family leave policies, and academic promotions.[20]

WOMEN IN PLASTIC SURGERY

The Women Plastic Surgeons Forum within the ASPRS was established in 1992. Organizing began as early as 1979 when Ann Riley, MD, organized a women's luncheon at the ASPS annual meeting. Participants decided not to organize a formal group at that time. Early participants believe that informal lunches continued, but not until 1992 did a formal group, the Women's Plastic Surgery Caucus, appear. The ASPRS supported the establishment of this women's group, some feel, primarily in response to the crisis over the safety of silicone breast implants. ASPRS support for the women's group may have anticipated the public relations benefit of women speaking to the health of women patients in response to the furor raised by these implants. Serving as an advocacy group gave women members a voice without requiring any ASPRS expense. In 1995, the women's group organized a "retreat," which formally became the Women's Plastic Surgery Forum, in 2003. The first woman to hold a major ASPS leadership role was Mary McGrath, MD, elected president of the PS Research Council in 1995. Roxanne Guy, MD, was the first woman elected to the ASPS Presidency in 2007, at the same time that Carolyn Kerrigan, MD, became the second woman to lead the Research Council. In the years before this, the Woman's Forum had organized an informal leadership coaching program, which they attribute to their success in breaking the glass ceiling. Wonderful oral interviews with some of these women leaders can be seen and heard through the Women Plastic Surgeons Forum.[21] These interviews provide an excellent narrative regarding the benefits that mutual support among women can have in creating leadership opportunities in a male-dominated society.

ORTHOPEDIC SURGERY

The Ruth Jackson Orthopedic Society (RJOS) was founded in 1983 as a support and networking group, with 42 initial members, growing to 1000 members in 2020.[22] One participant recalls that the meeting was held in secret, with many fearing to be labeled "feminists." Women-specific organizations can become a training ground for leadership as well as mentorship. Kristy L Weber, MD, FAAOS, and Past RJOS President, became the first woman to be president of the AAOS in 2020. In 2019, the RJOS reviewed what benefits came from past medical student scholarships given toward attending a meeting of the Society.[23] Of the 83 students who attended a meeting through this award between 2003 and 2016, 65 women (80%) recipients were either in the practice of orthopedics or in an orthopedic surgery residency. Further analysis showed that of the 49 student applicants whose application did not result in the scholarship, between 2014 and 2016, 22 (44.9%) were in an orthopedic program. Applicants for the RJOS scholarship clearly have an early interest in orthopedic surgery. The high "return rate" of student mentorship is reflected in similar programs within other women's professional organizations, such as the Women in Neurosurgery (WINS) or the Association of Women Surgeons who have similar programs and successes. Orthopedic surgery remains among the least representative surgical specialty, with less than 1% of all women residents participating in an orthopedic residency in the 2016 to 2017 academic year. The proportion of female residents within the field (14%) represents a small increase over the 11% found 10 years earlier during the 2005 to 2006 academic year. Among medical school faculty, only 17% of orthopedists are female, the lowest percentage among all other surgical specialties. Women comprise 6.5% of the membership of the AAOS. In academia, 8.7% of professors of orthopedic surgery were women and there was only 1 woman department chair.[24]

WOMEN IN NEUROSURGERY

The WINS held their first official meeting in 1990 led by Deborah Benzil, MD, at a time when there were less than 30 board-certified women neurosurgeons in the United States; most neurosurgery residencies had *never* trained a woman resident; only 5 training programs had women on the neurosurgery faculty. Dr Benzil describes how this first meeting evolved during a resident luncheon held during the national annual meeting: "I found my way to an empty table toward the back of the room when the miracle happened-another woman joined me at the table! Before I could say yes, yet another woman appeared. I can't speak for the others but I couldn't wait for the honored guest to finish talking. Truly remarkable to be in the company of 2 other female neurosurgeons. The program ended; the men exited while the three of us chatted on-soon magnetically joined by several other women. We made the impromptu decision to meet for a drink and to invite any other female neurosurgeon we could. November 1, 1989 this small group gathered and made the brave decision to form organization-WINS." By December a directory of just 19 women, a newsletter, and a first meeting began to take shape. From the first official meeting in October 1990, the number grew to include 33 members. Initially this group kept its meeting secret, but it was recognized without the expected backlash from the all-male leadership of the AANS in 1994.

The number of women in neurosurgery residencies at the inception of the organization was less than 2%, but by 2000 they represented 10% of residents and the number of women who had become board certified tripled to 72. Significantly, the attrition rate, originally a quarter of women starting residency, declined to 17% during that decade. The careers of the 3 women who started WINS achieved professional success as well: Gail Rosseau, MD, became the first woman neurosurgeon elected to the AANS board and the first female officer of that board; Karin Muraszko, MD, became the first female neurosurgical department chair and first to lead several neurosurgical societies; and Deborah Benzil, MD, became the first female chair of the Council of State Neurological Societies.[25]

In the 2000s, much like the women in plastic surgery, WINS hired consultants to "teach effective strategies for enhancing motivation and setting goals for professional development and personal achievement." In 2007, WINS inaugurated the Louise Eisenhardt MD Lecture, in honor of the woman who led Harvey Cushing's research team in the first half of the twentieth century. Dr Eisenhardt (1891–1967) managed Cushing's brain collection, establishing a unique record of neuropathology, and was the first editor of the Journal of Neurosurgery from its inception in 1944 until her retirement in 1966.

In 2008, with the encouragement of the AANS, WINS published a white paper that called for increasing female representation in neurosurgery, setting a goal of 20% females in training programs and among faculty by 2020.[26] In 2018, Shelly D Timmons, MD, PhD, became the first female neurosurgeon to be president of the AANS, 80 years after Louise Eisenhardt! Celebrating their 30th anniversary, WINS membership is approaching 700, and in 2018, achieved their resident goal of 20% representation. Programs sponsored by WINS have included the annual Eisenhardt lecture, scholarships for visiting international scholars, a regularly published WINS newsletter, near parity in scientific programming for AANS, and multiple programs during the year designed to promote and support women in neurosurgery.

WOMEN IN THORACIC SURGERY

Women in Thoracic Surgery (WTS) was founded in 1986. Between 1961 when the first 3 women were certified by the American Board of Thoracic Surgeons (ABTS) and 1980, that number had reached 10 (20 years later!). The most prominent woman in the specialty was Nina Starr Braunwald, MD, who became the first woman member of the American Association for Thoracic Surgery (AATS) in 1967 and the only one until 1989. Like many other women's surgical specialty organizations, WTS began as an informal breakfast gathering at the annual meetings of the AATS and the Society of Thoracic Surgeons (STS). These gatherings were organized by Leslie Kohman, MD. The group formalized in 1986. Early membership was facilitated by the American Board of Thoracic Surgery, which provided a list of women certified in the specialty. By 1989 there were a total of 89 ABTS women diplomats and 84 members of WTS, then called Women in Cardiothoracic Surgery (15 op cite). The organization continued to meet semiannually through the 1990s at luncheons held in connection with AATS and STS meetings. In 2000, at the 36th Annual Meeting of the STS, the WTS, and STS cohosted the WTS Symposium, marking the 15th anniversary of WTS. "The WTS Symposium was an important moment in the history of the WTS because it established a forum for celebrating the accomplishments of women in cardiothoracic surgery and recognized some of the hurdles that partially remain to date and also exemplified the growing support and recognition from male colleagues."[27] In 2000 there were 96 women certified by the ABTS, increasing to 309 women, 27% of board-certified thoracic surgeons by 2010. The WTS initiated student scholarships in 2005, awarding 67 through 2015. These fund programs for student travel to meetings, or rotations with women surgeons who may be mentors and have been successful enough to gain the support of the STS as well. As part of their outreach, the WTS has also established a robust social media presence supporting members and providing educational opportunities for students, fellows, and patients. Many firsts were accomplished in the third decade of the WTS. Dr Carolyn Reed became the first woman to chair the board of the ABTS in 2005 and was the first president of the Southern Thoracic Surgery Society (STSS). She was elected the first female president of the STS in 2013 but unfortunately died before assuming office. Other members have become first women to serve as president of various international thoracic societies as well.

Of the 22 surgical specialties, a recent study by Altieri and colleagues[28] finds that cardiothoracic surgery is viewed as the least welcoming to women surgeons. In a responding editorial Jessica Luc, MD, describes the efforts by her institution, the Washington University School of Medicine, where an active program of recruitment and support have brought the balance of women and underrepresented minorities to 50% of their graduates over the past 6 years.[29] The current percentage of women in thoracic training programs remains at 20% overall, but the robust mentoring, financial support, and recently increased emphasis on leadership programs supported by WTS indicate that continued progress is likely.

WOMEN IN OMF

In January of 2019, a group of University of Michigan women OMFS residents, Drs Kelly Sayer, Karen Carver, and Sara Hinds Anderson, organized the first Women in OMFS Symposium, supported by their program chairman, Brent Ward, MD, DDS. A second meeting occurred the following year, only to see the third event, scheduled for the Massachusetts General Hospital in Boston, canceled due to coronavirus disease 2019. During the 2019 annual meeting of the

AAOMS, a submitted abstract discussed results of a survey conducted at the second annual Women in Oral and Maxillofacial Surgery Leadership Symposium.[30] Attendees identified a significant lack of mentors (46%), sponsors (93%), or female colleagues (32.9%) in OMF as among the most significant barriers in their careers. These efforts represent a foundation for change in the specialty's gendered evolution. In 2018, Stephanie J Drew DMD, FACS, became the first woman elected to the presidency of the American College or Oral and Maxillofacial Surgeons (ACOMS). As the 26th president, her inaugural address summarized the achievements by women in her profession over the preceding 100 years.[31] In describing the career paths of 5 pioneering women dentists, Drew explicitly addresses the continued significant gender disparity within the dental field, and OMS specifically, and issued a call for transparency in resident, faculty, state society boards, AAOMS, and ABOMS boards. She also called for facilitating the development of increased diversity among all these organizations. Drew celebrates the women who currently hold leadership positions: 4 chairs of departments, several program directors, one Dean of students, and several full-time academicians. Yet, ACOMS (2018), with its 2655 members, has only 250 women members, of which 152 are residents. Drew calls out gender bias within the profession, citing previous studies exposing gender bias among practicing male OMS attending as well as residents, noting that contact by such individuals may discourage dental students from considering a career in OMF.[32] Drew also calls out the investigators of a survey demonstrating gender bias and sexual harassment issues within the profession. The investigators concluded that "A woman required a thick skin to sustain the indignity of gender bias and sexual harassment."[32] Drew, rightly condemns this "Regardless of the skin thickness, this is unacceptable and against the law. Period." The women in OMF have only recently begun to organize a distinct advocacy group. Evidence of the lack of opportunity for women in OMFS can be found in publication rates for women as opposed to men, which have not changed in more than 20 years.[33] In his 2010 article Laskin states, "Time commitment and social compromises remain the largest deterrents for women entering the specialty of OMFS."[34] Rostami and Laskin (33 op cite) report on the significant bias against women expressed by existing male members of the AAOMS; this stimulated a brisk letters to the editor response from several women members of the AAOMS. Laskin's view that hildbearing has a role in the discussion of female uitability for the OMFS profession returns to the rguments used in the 1800s against women ntering the professions. Stavropoulous, Delsol, nd Freedburg rightly call out the misogyny ised to deflect responsibly by the men address-ng the gender gap.[35] In his response Dr Laskin[36] ails to recognize that female fertility is not the ssue, but rather is a function of the failure to establish family-friendly norms within institutions hat constitutes the barrier. Again, addressing he issue in 2014 Natalie Eden notes that her own experience has been positive, with male nentors and sponsors, but her experience is not hared by all as seen in Sayers' study (13 op ite). Despite evidence to the contrary, Laskin in '015 denies the existence of bias against women n the profession pointing out that women are apable of performing OMS only to go on to 1ote that the "desire of some women to eventu-lly raise a family" remains an impediment to an cademic career. However, he does suggest hat academic institutions need to support amily-friendly initiatives, such as university-ased child care services, a sign of an evolution n attitude.[37]

There are significant benefits to a specific Woman in OMFS" organization; this creates the opportunities for mutual support, mentorship, nd sponsorship like those that have existed mong other women's groups since the nine-eenth century. A women's association can direct efforts to reduce the barriers that still exist, advo-ate for better policies, as well as work to increase epresentation and inclusion. In 2016, Kolokytha nd Miloro[38] examined the forces that encourage vomen to enter academic OMFS, finding that nvolvement with students, research potential, nd the avoidance of the business side of practice vere significant in the decision to enter academia. The investigators' recommendation to increase nvolvement included improved mentorship, and ncreased contact with other female OMF sur-geons confirms this argument.[38] The current ess-formal meetings being held are a valuable first step. Despite the cancellation of the planned 2020 Women in OMFS Symposium, the residents sec-tion of AAOMS have started a mentorship program natching resident mentors to dental student nentees, assisting them in their OMFS residency application process.

SUMMARY

Women's groups have played a valuable role in promoting women's greater participation in their specialty organizations. In her presidential address, to the Southeastern Surgical Congress, Rebecca Britt, MD, highlighted the importance of these organizations in providing both mentorship and sponsorship. Mentorship involves being a role model to teach, guide, and advise the novice, a kind of counselor. Sponsorship involves sup-porting the participation and promotion of the novice within the power structure, serving as an advocate. The gender of the mentor or sponsor is not inherently important, but such support struc-tures are less available for women within the surgi-cal community than they are to men.[39] The role of the women's associations in their specialty as-sumes critical importance during the training years and beyond. The AWS' recently published "#HeForShe Task Force" offers explicit guidelines for reducing implicit bias, and the American Surgi-cal Association (ASA) has produced a white paper with recommendations to address issues of eq-uity, diversity, and inclusion.[40,41] These 2 papers outline a detailed strategy that can be adopted if a genuine interest in increasing diversity, inclusion, and equity is sincerely held. Chapman and col-leagues[42] looked at the factors predicting women's representation in GME. The investigators found that having female faculty and having them participate in the third year clinical curriculum correlated strongly with women students entering those fields.[42] In July 2020, the American Board of Medical Specialties (ABMS) established a new policy on parental leave, adopted from the ACGME recommendations of the previous year. These 2 powerful forces in postgraduate medical education acknowledge the necessity of family-friendly policies.[43] Specific recommendations for enhancing women's opportunities within surgery include simple strategies: minimizing evening and weekend meetings, addressing disruptive behavior, reviewing policies for recruitment and retention, and nominating women for positions within and without the department or institution.[44] The women's specialty organizations have pro-vided a pathway to leadership for their members that are still relatively scarce within their wider pro-fessional associations.

The University of Michigan, by sponsoring the Women in OMFS meetings, and the example of the diverse nature of the faculty and residents at the University of North Carolina, demonstrate that gender attention and diversity are possible only when there is a willingness within the institu-tions to promote them. And that, when there is some diversity, there will be more. As one observer stated, "When applicants interview and see the di-versity of faculty and residents---they are more likely to rank us higher than a program such as--- are all white males."

The history of women in medicine and dentistry reveals striking parallels as women overcame significant resistance and forged paths toward professional inclusion and success, seeking education, community acceptance, and bonds with their fellow professionals. Women joined suffrage activists and served women and children as their primary patients. However, full inclusion and participation remained then and now, elusive. Women-based surgical subspecialty organizations provide abundant leadership, speaking, and mentoring opportunities. The surgical specialties examined here represent some of the older and more established such organizations. These specialties provide a model that should be useful, as the women in OMS increase representation within their profession, their academic institutions, and their organizations and bring to their organizations genuinely valued diversity, inclusion, and equity. Achieving gender parity requires a robust commitment if more than slight incremental improvement will occur.

ACKNOWLEDGMENT

The author thank Roberta Gartside, MD, Susan Zhong, MD, Margaret Skiles, MD, for plastic surgery; Eugene Braunwald, Leslie Kohman, MD, and Allison Goldfine, MD, for thoracic surgery; Leslie Anderson, MD, for orthopedic surgery; Deborah Benzil for neurosurgery; and Lorenza Donnelly, DDS; Eve Bluestein, DDS MD, and Franci Stavropoulis, DDS, for their comments on oral maxillosfacial surgery.

DISCLOSURE

The authors have nothing to disclose.

REFERENCES

1. Campbell KI, McCammon HJ. Elizabeth Blackwell's Heirs: Women as Physicians in the United States 1880-1930. Work Occup 2005;32(3):290–318.
2. U.S. Department of Health and Human Services, Health Resources and Services Administration, National Center for Health Workforce Analysis. 2017. Sex, Race, and Ethnic Diversity of U.S, Health Occupations (2011-2015). Rockville, Maryland.
3. Rosenberg GN. The 1964 Civil Rights Ace: the crucial role of social movements in the enactment and implementation of anti-discrimination law. St Louis U L J 2004;49:441–2.
4. Haug JN. A review of women in surgery. Bull Am Coll Surg 1975;60(9):21–3.
5. Nakayam DK. Pioneering women in American Pediatric Surgery. J Ped Surg 2018;53(11):2361–8.
6. Fitzgerald C, Smith R, Xian L-O, et al. Screening for Harassment, Abuse and Discrimination among Surgery Residents: An EAST Multicenter Trial. Am Surg 2019;85(5):456–61.
7. Kinsler MS. The American Woman Dentist: A Brief Historical Review from 1855 through 1968. Bull Hist Dent 1969;17(2):25–31.
8. Drachman VG. Limits of Progress: The professional Lives of Women Doctors, 1881-1926. Bull Hist Med 1986;60:58–72.
9. Bennet CL, Baker O, Rangel EL, et al. The Gender Gap in Surgical Residencies. JAMA Surg 2020;155(9):893–4.
10. Surdu S, Mertz E, Langelier M. Dental Workforce Trends: a national study of gender diversity and practice patterns. Medical Care Research and Review 2020. Available at: https://journals.sagepub.com/doi/full/10.1177/1077558720952667. Accessed December 1, 2020.
11. Vujicic M, Yarborough C, Munsons M. Time to Talk About the Gender Gap in Dentist Earnings. JADA 2017;148(4):204–6.
12. Pennings I. Gender Diversity in Oral and Maxillofacial Surgery. Contour 2018;2(7):14–7.
13. Eden N. How will Women Shape the Future of Oral and Maxillofacial Surgery?. Available at: https://cdn.ymaws.com/www.acoms.org/resource/resmgr/awards/Natalie_Eden_Essay.pdf. Accessed December 22, 2020.
14. Abdel Aziz H, DuCoin C, Welsh DJ, et al. 2018 ACS Governors Survey: Gender inequality and harassment remain a challenge in surgery. Bull Am Coll Surg 2019;104:21–30.
15. Kohman LJ, Hoefer JM. The Formation and Function of women's groups within specialty societies. J Am Med Womens Assoc 1991;46(3):92–4.
16. Stern V. Few women in top Posts Despite Gains in Overall Ranks. Gen Surg News 2016. Available at: https://www.generalsurgerynews.com/Article/PrintArticle?articleID=37814. Accessed December 26, 2020.
17. Lillemoe KD, Ahrendt GM, Yeo CJ, et al. Surgery: Still an "old boys' club"? Surgery 1994;116:255–9 [discussion: 259].
18. Available at: https://www.womensurgeons.org/page/AboutAWS and https://www.womensurgeons.org/page/History (Accessed December 23, 2020.
19. Saamia S, Juliet E, Geeta L, et al. The Association of Women Surgeons Research Grant: An Analysis of the first 25 Years. Am J Surg 2020;220(5):1146–50.
20. Schneideman DS. Women at the Helm of the ACS: Charting a course of gender equity 2018. Available at: https://bulletin.facs.org/2018/09/women-at-the-helm-of-the-acs-charting-a-course-to-gender-equity/. Accessed December 2, 2020.
21. Available at: https://www.plasticsurgery.org/for-medical-professionals/community/women-plastic-surgeons-forum. (Accessed December 21, 2020)

22. Available at: http://www.rjos.org/(Accessed Dec 26, 2020.

23. Sravya B, Cannada Lisa K, Julia Balch S. What Proportion of Women Who Received Funding to Attend a Ruth Jackson Orthopaedic Society Meeting Pursued a Career in Orthopaedics? Clin Orthop Relat Res 2019;477:1722–6.

24. Chambers CC, Ihnow SB, Monroe EJ, et al. Women in Orthopaedic Surgery: Population Trends in Trainees and Practicing Surgeons. J Bone Joint Surg Am 2018;100(17):e116.

25. Hdeib A, Elder T, Krivosheya D, et al. History of Women in Neurosurgery (WINS). Neurosurg Focus 2021;50(3):E16.

26. Benzil DL, Abosch A, Germano I, et al. The future of neurosurgery: a white paper on the recruitment and retention of women in neurosurgery. J Neurosurg 2008;109:378–86.

27. Antonoff Mara B, David Elizabeth A, Donington Jessica S, et al. Women in thoracic surgery: 30 years history. Ann Thorac Surg 2016;101(1):399–409.

28. Altieri M, Price K, Yang J, et al. What are women being advised by mentors when applying to surgery? Am Surg 2020;86(3):266–72.

29. Luc JGY, Preventza O, Moon MR, et al. Keep the Pipeline Open for Women Applying to Cardiothoracic Surgery. Am Surg 2020. https://doi.org/10.1177/0003134820951478. 3134820951478.

30. Sayre K, Carver KZ, Anderson S, et al. Barriers to Women in Oral and Maxillofacial Surgery: A Cross Sectional Survey. 2019;77(9 supplement E53) Available at: https://doi.org/10.1016/j.joms.2019.06.070. Accessed January 3, 2020.

31. Available at: https://www.acoms.org/news/407850/2023671182. Accessed December 21, 2020.

32. Rostami F, Laskin D. Male perception of women in oral and Maxillofacial Surgery. J Oral Maxillofac Surg 2014;72:2383–5.

33. Consky Elizabeth K, Bradshaw Shenan M, Wein Alexander N, et al. The proportion of female authors in oral and maxillofacial surgery literature has not changed in 20 years. J Oral Maxillofac Surg 2020;78:877–81.

34. Rostami F, Ahmed AE, Best AM, et al. The changing personal and professional characteristics of women in oral and maxillofacial surgery. J Oral Maxillofac Surg 2010;68(2):381–5.

35. Letters to the Editor. J Oral Maxillofac Surg 2015;73(6):1024–5.

36. Letter to the EditorJ. Laskin DM. Oral Maxillofac Surg 2015;73(6):1026.

37. Laskin DM. The role of women in academic oral and maxillofacial surgery. J Oral Maxillofac Surg 2015;73(4):579.

38. Kolokytha A, Miloro M. Why do women choose to enter Academic Oral and maxillofacial Surgery? J Oral Maxillofac Surg 2016;74(5):881–8.

39. Rebecca B. Membership matters: reclaiming the joy in surgery. Am Surg 2020;86(7):725–9.

40. DiBrito SR, Lopez CM, Jones C, et al. Reducing Implicit Bias: Association of Women Surgeons #HeForShe Task Force Best Practice Recommendations. J Am Coll Surg 2019;228(3):303–9.

41. West MA, Hwang S, Maier RV, et al. Ensuring equity, diversity, and inclusion in academic surgery. Ann Surg 2018;268(3):403–7.

42. Chapman CH, Hwang WT, Wang X, et al. Factors that predict for representation of women in physician graduate medical education. Med Educ Online 2019;24(1):1624132.

43. Available at: https://www.abms.org/news-events/abms-announces-progressive-leave-policy-for-residents-and-fellows. Accessed September 12, 2020.

44. Amalia C, Leigh N. Breaking Down the Walls: Removing Structural Barriers for Women in Academic Surgery. Am Surg 2011;77(11):1437.

Trends in Diversity Related to Gender and Race in the Surgical Specialties and Subspecialties Inclusive of Oral and Maxillofacial Surgery

Brett L. Ferguson, DDS, FACD, FICD[a],*, Maria Morgan, JD[b], Susan B. Wilson, PhD, MBA[c]

KEYWORDS

- Gender discrimination • Racial discrimination • Diversity • Underrepresentation
- Surgical residencies

KEY POINTS

- Medical training in Kansas City during the 1950s and at the University of Kansas School of Medicine was segregated and separate.
- Legal cases associated with affirmative action including Grutter v Bollinger, Regents of the University of California v Bakke, and the Flexner report are discussed.
- Women and minorities involved with surgery and surgery training, with the concept of equity, diversity, and inclusion are defined.
- The demographics of surgical training related to gender, racial, and ethnic diversity of trainees are reviewed.

In Kansas City, Missouri during the 1950s, the hospital system was segregated and separate; the medical professionals were trained separately, and patients typically were maintained by their race-based medical personnel. The University of Kansas was an academic medical center (AMC) that dominated the medical fabric of our local community and is still considered today a major AMC. It was in Kansas City and the exposure to a 2-tiered medical system that led to the revelation by a family member, Dr John Ramos (**Fig. 1**) and the first African American (AA) to achieve specialty-based certification in Radiology, of the effects of discrimination as it affected our family[1] as well as my personal mentor, Dr Carl Peterson, MD, and general surgeon. Dr Peterson started the first AA specialty physician group west of the Mississippi (Dr John Ramos was a partner; Dr Carl M. Peterson Collection AC029 http:///black-archives.org>files) in the Kansas City metropolitan area and helped the transformation of the segregated system of medical training to one of integration at General House Hospital/Truman Medical Center/University of Missouri–Kansas City School of Medicine.[2] I had the opportunity to meet a giant during this era, Donald Sheffield Ferguson, who was the second AA to graduate from University of Kansas School of Medicine (KU SOM) in 1942 (KU History 1938 by Nancy Hulston). He set up practice in Kansas City, Missouri as a dermatologist, was active in civil rights, and died in 1989. In addition, the first female graduate (1958) from

a Department of Oral and Maxillofacial Surgery, Truman Medical Center, 2301 Holmes, Kansas City, MO 64108, USA; b Department of Diversity and Inclusion, Truman Medical Center, 2301 Holmes, Kansas City, MO 64108, USA; c Department of Diversity and Inclusion, UMKC School of Dentistry, 650 E. 25th Street, Kansas City, MO 64108, USA
* Corresponding author.
E-mail address: Brett.ferguson@tmcmed.org

Oral Maxillofacial Surg Clin N Am 33 (2021) 491–503
https://doi.org/10.1016/j.coms.2021.07.001
1042-3699/21/© 2021 Elsevier Inc. All rights reserved.

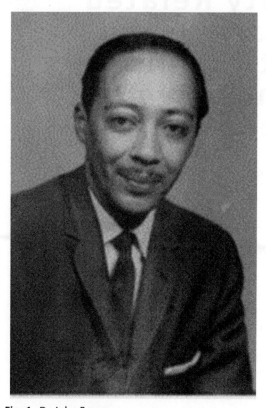

Fig. 1. Dr John Ramos.

the KU SOM was Marjorie Cates (hematology) (and a family member) (**Fig. 2**).[3]

The Grutter v Bollinger 539 US 306 (2003) (**Fig. 3**)[4] and the Regents of the University of California v Bakke (1978) were 2 legal cases that were landmark cases concerning affirmative action in student admissions, well known in the Kansas City metropolitan area. The ramification from these 2 cases favors underrepresented minority groups in the admissions process but does not violate the Fourteenth Amendment Clause so long as it takes into account other evaluative factors in admission. The use of race in admissions decisions to further a compelling interest in obtaining the educational benefits that flow from a diverse student body was now law.

Gender discrimination, like racial discrimination, is a social process whereby individuals are treated differently BUT disadvantageously, under similar circumstances, on the basis of gender.[5] The interesting concept of gender discrimination was seen early, and even in 1970, women only comprised less than 6%[6] of any medical school in the United States or Canada. The year 2017, a very good year as it relates to women, revealed for the first time that more women than men were enrolled in medical school. This increase is not being felt downstream, as the American Surgical Association,

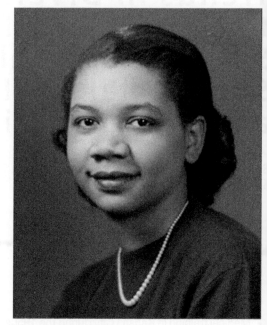

Fig. 2. Dr Marjorie Cates.

American College of Surgeons (ACS), the American Medical Association (AMA), the Association of American Medical Colleges, and the Accreditation Council for Graduate Medical Education (ACGME) all have produced extensive reports on the underrepresentation of women and racial minorities in the medical profession relative to their numbers in the general population (**Fig. 4**).[7] Louis Sullivan, MD, Section of Health and Human Services during G.H.W. Bush administration, wrote in 2010 about the 1910 Flexner Report.[8,9]

The Flexner Report[8] was a book-length synopsis on the state of medical education in the United States and Canada, under the aegis of the Carnegie Foundation. This report ultimately recommended the closure of a large consortium of medical schools. Abraham Flexner's Carnegie Foundation Bulletin No. 4.[10] The report led to high-quality standards and training, but amid these times, significant energy for women demanding equality, and worker safety/working conditions, and discrimination were a part of the social fabric of life. Disparities were noted to exist in areas of gender, race, ethnicity, age, socioeconomic factors, and access and were unhindered by government action. A byproduct of the Flexner Report was closure of 5 out of 7 predominantly black medical schools, and an unspoken mandate for American Universities to revert to male-only admittance to "accommodate" a smaller admission pool. It should be remembered that universities had started to evolve in the mid to latter part of the nineteenth century to open and expand female

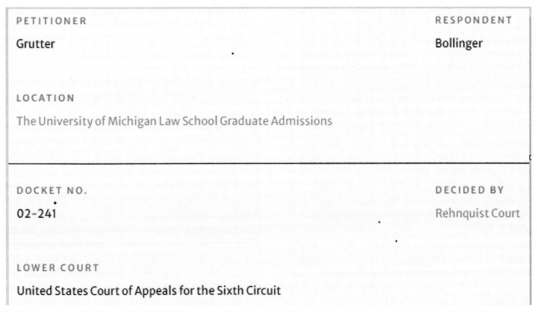

PETITIONER	RESPONDENT
Grutter	Bollinger

LOCATION

The University of Michigan Law School Graduate Admissions

DOCKET NO.	DECIDED BY
02-241	Rehnquist Court

LOWER COURT

United States Court of Appeals for the Sixth Circuit

Fig. 3. Grutter v Bollinger 503 US 306 Supreme Court of US. (*Used with* permission from Oyez (https://www.oyez.org), a free law project by Justia and the Legal Information Institute of Cornell Law School.)

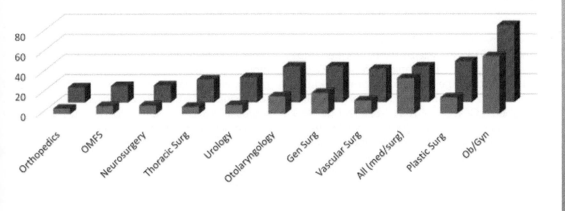

Fig. 4. Lee and colleagues residency interview experiences in oral and maxillofacial surgery differ by gender and affect residency ranking. Female residents and practitioners stratified by specialty in 2018 (source: American Association of Oral and Maxillofacial Surgeons Directory 2017 to 2018; American Association of Medical Colleges [AAMC] 2017 Active Practicing Surgeons by Specialty; AAMC 2017 to 2018 Residents by Specialty). Gen, general; med/surg, medical/surgical; Ob/Gyn, obstetrics/gynecology; OMFS, oral-maxillofacial surgery; Surg, surgery. (*From* Lee JS, Ji YD, Kushner H, Kaban LB, Peacock ZS. Residency Interview Experiences in Oral and Maxillofacial Surgery Differ by Gender and Affect Residency Ranking. J Oral Maxillofac Surg. 2019 Nov;77(11):2179-2195.)

admissions. Oberlin College, Vassar, and Pembroke Colleges certainly come to mind. It is of interest that Oberlin College is the second oldest continuously operating coeducational institute of higher learning in the world (Oberlin History Oberlin College and Conservatory, February 2017). In 1835, Oberlin was one of the first colleges to admit AA, and, in 1837, the first to admit women.[11,12] Vassar College (founded in 1861) was the second degree-granting institution of higher learning for women in the United States (part of the historic Seven Sisters liberal arts colleges). The number of women in 1970 revealed less than 6% comprising classes in medical school and less than 2% of the ACS college membership in 1975 (**Table 1**).[5,6,13]

Women have been involved with surgery throughout human history.[6,14] Debrah Wirtzfeld[15] wrote of western civilization that the earliest account of female surgeons dates to 3500 BCE, with Queen Shubad of Ur (also referred to as Puabi; Royal Cemetery at Ur Iraq). Queen Shubad of Ur's tomb was found with buried surgical instruments. Dr James Barry was a nineteenth century surgeon who was in actuality a woman, Dr Miranda Stewart, and was the first qualified British surgeon and a military surgeon. The first female physicians in North America were Drs Elizabeth Blackwell and Emily Jennings Stowe (Stowe learned about women suffrage from Susan B. Anthony) in the 1860s; the first female surgeons were Dr Mary Edwards Walker (a dedicated advocate for the abolition of slavery and for women's rights and was the first military female surgeon), and Jennie Smillie Robertson (the first female surgeon in Canada, and first to perform major gynecologic surgery) (Clinical Congress 2019 Special Session, Women Pioneers in Surgery).[14] Dr Matilda Arabella Evans, considered to be the first underrepresented minority woman surgeon, attended and graduated from Oberlin College in 1891, received her MD in 1897, practiced surgery for interracial patients in South Carolina, practiced Obstetrics/Gynecology and Surgery,[16] and established St. Luke's Hospital, which operated a school of nursing. Today, St. Luke's School of Nursing is the oldest hospital-based, diploma school in continuous operation. In addition, Dr Evans raised 11 orphan children! Dr Dorothy Lavinia Brown (**Fig. 5**) graduated from Meharry Medical college in 1948, became the first AA woman to be inducted into the ACS in 1959, and was the first AA woman to be elected to the Tennessee General Assembly (Changing the face of Medicine https://cfmedicine.nlm.nih.gov/phycians/biography-46.html).[14,17]

Dr James Durham, born into slavery in 1762, was able to buy his freedom and began his medical practice in New Orleans. The first AA to earn a medical degree was Dr James McCune Smith in 1837, graduating from the University of Glasgow, followed by Dr David Jones Peck, the first AA to graduate from a US medical school (Rush Medical College) in 1847. Almost 20 years later, Dr Rebecca Lee Crumpler was the first AA woman to receive her MD in 1864. It was in 1867 that Robert Tanner Freeman was one of the first 6 graduates in dental medicine from Harvard University, becoming the first AA to receive a dental degree from an American medical school. In 1973, Patricia Bath was the first AA to complete a residency in Ophthalmology and in 1988 was the first AA female physician to receive a medical patent for her Laserphaco Probe (for cataract treatment). Dr Patrice Harris (**Fig. 6**) became President of the AMA in 2019, as the first AA woman to achieve the top leadership position (Duke University: Chronology of Achievements for Black History Month: A Medical Perspective).

From the above perspective, the concept of ensuring equity, diversity, and inclusion in surgery and the surgical subspecialties is and has been distant (**Table 2**).

Data now should include not only information on undergraduate medicine and dentistry but also statistics on postsecondary education trends, as this flow of students should reflect the demographics of our current US population. For the year 2017 to 2018,[18] this study found that black and Hispanic students are underrepresented at more selective universities by 6 percentage points, and black students are overrepresented in the for-profit college sector by 15 percentage points. White and Asian students are overrepresented at more selective colleges by 4 to 8 percentage points. Native Americans were consistently overrepresented at public 2-year colleges and underrepresented at 4-year colleges (2009–2017). Pacific Islanders representation declined at 2-year and were overrepresented at 4-year for-profit colleges (2009–2017). If the pipeline for professional schools (US Medical and Dental schools) is made of this cohort, then diversity may be problematic. Koka and colleagues[19] published as a commentary a review of leadership diversity in dentistry (**Fig. 7**). Their leadership review revealed that one-half of the 12 dental specialties have not elevated a single non-white person to the office of president, and one had neither a non-white person nor a woman hold this position. Interestingly, the American College of Dentists (ACD) celebrated the Presidency of Juliann Bluitt Foster as the first AA and woman of the American

Table 1
Percentage of women of US medical school graduates and applicants to accreditation council for graduate medical education-accredited surgical residency programs and fellowship programs from 2008 to 2018

Characteristic	Initial	Final	P Value	χ^2
US graduating class				
Total, no.	15,227	19,533	NA	NA
Female, no. (%)	7028 (46)	9260 (47)	<.001	15.44
Integrated vascular				
Total, no.	112	392	NA	NA
Female, no. (%)	18 (16)	106 (27)	.001	10.33
Integrated thoracic				
Total, no.	63	185	NA	NA
Female, no. (%)	8 (13)	50 (27)	<.001	18.31
Integrated plastic surgery				
Total, no.	332	527	NA	NA
Female, no. (%)	109 (33)	182 (35)	.58	0.30
Neurosurgery				
Total, no.	459	423	NA	NA
Female, no. (%)	74 (16)	91 (22)	.19	1.71
Otolaryngology				
Total, no.	684	730	NA	NA
Female, no. (%)	202 (30)	242 (33)	.51	0.44
Orthopedics				
Total, no.	1360	1387	NA	NA
Female, no. (%)	193 (14)	226 (16)	.003	8.77
Urology				
Total, no.	532	462	NA	NA
Female, no. (%)	130 (24)	128 (28)	.03	4.61
General surgery (categorical)				
Total, no.	4429	4261	NA	NA
Female, no. (%)	1211 (27)	1636 (38)	<.001	188.41
Vascular fellowship				
Total, no.	131	126	NA	NA
Female, No. (%)	24 (18)	38 (30)	.09	2.85
Thoracic fellowship				
Total, no.	103	122	NA	NA
Female, no. (%)	14 (13)	32 (26)	.06	3.53
Plastic surgery fellowship				
Total, no.	342	122	NA	NA
Female, no. (%)	111 (32)	47 (39)	.08	3.14
Pediatric fellowship				
Total, no.	64	82	NA	NA
Female, no. (%)	32 (50)	44 (54)	.002	9.43
Colorectal fellowship				
Total, no.	113	130	NA	NA
Female, no. (%)	32 (28)	57 (44)	.03	5.03

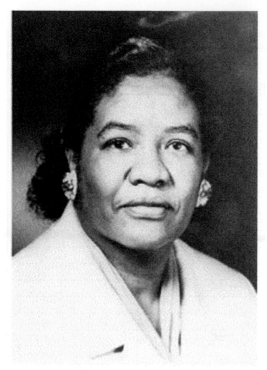

Fig. 5. Dr Dorothy Brown. (*From* Ali AM, McVay CL. Women in Surgery: A History of Adversity, Resilience, and Accomplishment. J Am Coll Surg. 2016 Oct;223(4):670-3.)

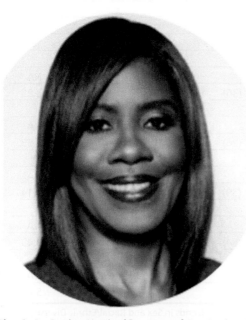

Fig. 6. Dr Patrice Harris. (*Courtesy of* Dr. Patrice A. Harris; used with permission.)

College of Dentistry in 1994,[20] and the first elected AA man of the ACD was Leo Rouse, in 2021. This should and must be recognized as not being optimal and should stimulate a need to take action. Pipeline diversification of our workforce is tied to diversification of student body but will not mimic the US population overall in reality. However, this should be a goal.

The demographics of the United States are changing, and the racial and ethnic diversities are increasing. For the year July 1, 2019, the population of the United States was 328,256,523.[21] The race breakdown was white alone, 76.3%; white alone, not Hispanic or Latino, 60.1%; Hispanic, 18.5%; black, 13.4%; Asian alone, 5.9%; American Indian and Alaska Native, 1.3% (US Census.gov July 1, 2019). In 2019, the female percentage in the United States was 50.8%. In 2016, a greater percentage of undergraduates was women than men across all racial/ethnic groups (Status and Trends in the Education of Racial and Ethnic Groups 2018; NCES 2019-028 US Department of Education). The gap between female and male enrollment was widest for black students at 62% versus 38% and lowest for Asians at 53% versus 47%. The American Dental Educators Association (ADEA) report for the current enrollment for all SODs for 2019 revealed the following: total enrollment of 6231 students, with 3273 women (52.5%) and 2952 men (47.4%).[22] In this cohort, the racial breakdown is as follows: white, 3114 (50%); Asian, 1426 (22.9%); Hispanic, 623 (10%); blacks, 360 (5.8%) and American Indian, 5 (.01%). Looking at trends related to US medical students by the American Association of Medical Colleges[23,24], the number of matriculants was 21,326. Conclusions revealed that white male and female individuals decreased; black, Hispanic, and Alaska Native remain underrepresented among medical school matriculants. Review of physician workforce numbers for 2019 (**Fig. 8**)[13–31] reveals a total of 936,254, with 63.7% men versus 36.3 women (represents 340,018 individuals). Racial numbers of this workforce is as follows: whites, 56.2%; Asian, 17.1%; Hispanic, 5.8%; blacks, 5.0%; and American Indian, 0.3% (**Fig. 9**).

The workforce numbers for dentistry in 2020 (ADA Health Policy Supply of Dentists in the US: 2001-2020) reveals 201,117 individuals, and women represent 34.5%, which is 69,385 individuals. Racial numbers for the dental workforce are as follows: white, 70.2%; Asian, 18%; Hispanic, 5.9%; and black, 3.8%. In summation, the medical and dental workforces do not reflect the US population in terms of racial disparity.

Table 2
Trends in underrepresented racial/ethnic minorities of US medical school graduates and applicants to accreditation council for graduate medical education-accredited surgical residency programs and fellowship programs from 2008 to 2018

Characteristic	Asian			Black			Hispanic			White		
	No. (%)	P Value	Change[a]	No. P9	P Value	Change[a]	No. (%)	P Value	Change[a]	No. (%)	P Value	Change[a]
US graduating class												
Initial[b]	5524 (22)	.02	←	1113 (7)	<.001	→	1187 (8)	<.001	←	10,358 (68)	<.001	→
Final[c]	4660 (24)			1280 (6.5)			1760 (9)			12,186 (62)		
Integrated vascular												
Initial	32 (29)	<.001	→	6 (5)	.83	NS	22 (20)	<.001	→	47 (42)	.54	NS
Final	70 (18)			31 (8)			32 (8)			155 (40)		
Integrate thoracic												
Initial	18 (29)	<.001	→	2 (3)	.17	NS	5 (8)	.35	NS	25 (40)	.004	←
Final	34 (18)			12 (7)			11 (6)			75 (41)		
Integrated plastic surgery												
Initial	50 (15)	.06	NS	14 (4)	.25	NS	28 (8)	.61	NS	213 (64)	<.001	→
Final	105 (20)			36 (7)			49 (9)			242 (46)		
Neurosurgery												
Initial	95 (21)	<.001	→	41 (9)	.001	→	42 (9)	.20	NS	237 (52)	.18	NS
Final	86 (20)			22 (5)			34 (8)			184 (44)		
Otolaryngology												
Initial	167 (24)	.05	→	38 (6)	.93	NS	57 (8)	.61	NS	373 (55)	.007	→
Final	145 (20)			44 (6)			68 (9)			371 (51)		
Orthopedics												
Initial	201 (15)	.02	→	113 (8)	<.001	→	92 (7)	.09	NS	896 (66)	.15	NS
Final	108 (14)			83 (6)			107 (8)			863 (62)		
Urology												
Initial	113 (21)	.68	NS	38 (7)	<.001	→	32 (6)	.82	NS	311 (59)	.01	→
Final	93 (20)			20 (4)			35 (8)			258 (56)		
General surgery (categorical)												
Initial	1302 (29)	<.001	→	370 (8)	<.001	→	462 (10)	<.001	→	1959 (44.2)	<.001	←
Final	762 (18)			296 (7)			395 (9)			1886 (44.3)		

(continued on next page)

Table 2
(continued)

Characteristic	Asian			Black			Hispanic			White		
	No. (%)	P Value	Change[a]	No. P9	P Value	Change[a]	No. (%)	P Value	Change[a]	No. (%)	P Value	Change[a]
Vascular fellowship												
Initial	30 (23)	.87	NS	9 (7)	.23	NS	12 (9)	.36	NS	78 (60)	.02	→
Final	29 (23)			6 (5)			9 (7)			66 (52)		
Thoracic fellowship												
Initial	30 (28)	.18	NS	2 (4)	.55	NS	11 (10)	.04	→	69 (64)	.16	NS
Final	20 (16)			5 (4)			3 (3)			66 (54)		
Plastic surgery fellowship												
Initial	72 (21)	.31	NS	17 (5)	.81	NS	35 (10)	.14	NS	209 (61)	.18	NS
Final	31 (25)			6 (5)			8 (7)			65 (53)		
Pediatric fellowship												
Initial	11 (17)	.17	NS	5 (8)	.17	NS	6 (9)	.26	NS	36 (56)	.37	NS
Final	6 (7)			3 (4)			9 (11)			49 (60)		
Colorectal fellowship												
Initial	28 (25)	.002	→	6 (5)	.38	NS	9 (8)	.22	NS	58 (51)	.32	NS
Final	22 (17)			4 (3)			8 (6)			71 (55)		

[a] ↑, significant increase ($P<.05$); ↓, significant decrease ($P<.5$); NS, no significant change ($P≥.05$).

[b] All initial percentages calculated from data starting in 2008, except integrated thoracic (2009), plastic surgery (2010), and neurosurgery (2009).

[c] All final percentages calculated from data in 2018, except plastic surgery fellowship (2017).

From Choinski K, Lipsitz E, Indes J, Phair J, Gao Q, Denesopolis J, Koleilat I. Trends in Sex and Racial/Ethnic Diversity in Applicants to Surgery Residency and Fellowship Programs. JAMA Surg. 2020 Aug 1;155(8):778-781 with permission.

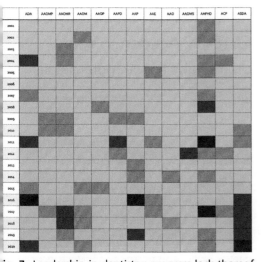

Fig. 7. Leadership in dentistry: progress lack thereof. Distribution of white woman (*light pink*), white man (*light blue*), nonwhite woman (*violet*), and nonwhite man (*dark blue*) presidents of dental associations from 2001 through 2020. AAE, American Association of Endodontists; AAO, American Association of Orthodontists; AAOM, American Academy of Oral Medicine; AAOMP, American Academy of Oral and Maxillofacial Pathology; AAOMR, American Academy of Oral and Maxillofacial Radiology; AAOP, American Academy of Orofacial Pain; AAP, American Academy of Periodontology; AAPD, American Academy of Pediatric Dentistry; AAPHD, American Association of Public Health Dentistry; ACP, American College of Prosthodontists; ADA, American Dental Association; ASDA, American Society of Dental Anesthesiologists. *From* Koka S, Phasuk K, Kattadiyil MT, Mutluay M. Leadership diversity in dentistry: Progress and lack thereof. J Am Dent Assoc. 2021 Feb;152(2):85-88.)

Looking at the number and percentage of ACGME learners (residents and fellows) reveals more inspiring numbers as they relate to gender diversification.[13,18,19,21,25–30] All specialties reveal a total number of 139,848 residents and fellows, 75,730 men (54.2%) and 64,118 women (45.8%), with the highest female numbers by percentage in Endocrinology, Neonatal Medicine, Obstetrics/Gynecology, and Pediatrics. The lowest percentages of women in resident specialty areas are Interventional Cardiology (13%), Neurosurgery (19.5), Orthopedic Surgery (16.0%), and Sports Medicine (12.9%). When looking at General Surgery (43.1%), Ophthalmology (41.2), Otolaryngology (38%), Plastic Surgery (40.9%), and Vascular Surgery (33.1%), the percentage of gender diversification is promising. However, these numbers do not tell the whole story, as less than one-third of surgeons globally are women, and women make up less than one-quarter of 10 surgical specialties (Physician Specialty Data Report 2020). Increasing diversity in graduating medical school classes may not and does not translate to increasing diversity in the surgical training applicant pool. Black women account for less than 3% of US doctors[31] (https://fortune.com/2020/08/09/health-care-rascism-black-women-doctors/). Benay and colleagues[32] found downstream issues as leadership positions from 22 major surgical organizations were less diverse relative to the surgical workforce and population, with only a 4% non-white representation. In fact, surgeons from underrepresented minorities in medicine (URM) account for 7% of Academic Surgery faculty. No increase in AA and a decrease in Hispanic academic surgery faculty occurred from 2005 to 2018. In 2019, there are 24 female chairs of surgery in the United States (AAMC Data 7-15-2019).[33–35]

American Association of Oral and Maxillofacial Surgeons (AAOMS) membership data (L. Rafetto, published data, 2017) specifically will be reviewed to compare with medical/dental student characteristics and trainee data. The Oral and Maxillofacial Surgeons (OMS) community contains both practicing and retired members, as well as resident members, totaling 10,342. Women are 629 of 6620 active members (10%), retired 48 of 2265 members (2%), and residents 306 of 1457 (21%) (**Fig. 10**).

Therefore, approximately 10% of the OMS membership is women. There are now 4 female Chairs of OMS Departments nationally for 2021, representing 100 programs (4%) (AAOMS Membership-Gender Comparison 2021). The OMS number of women in residency is 21% for 2021, but overall membership is low. The rationale for this is multifactorial (Lee, 2019; Burke, 2018 and Kyriaki, 2017)[22,24,36–40] and includes lack of mentorship, lack of role models, attraction to the work itself, perception that surgical life is not compatible with the disproportionate burden that women bear of caregiving responsibilities, sexual and covert harassment, and gender discrimination.[6,27,32,33,37,41,42] Attrition rates when female doctors pursue and are accepted into surgical training are higher (withdrawal or exclusion) with women perceiving a higher standard to enter and thrive in the surgical field.[31,43] As it relates to gender discrimination, medical students continue to report the most gender-based discrimination on surgery rotations.[36]

AAOMS leadership in 2021 has made a commitment to diversity and presently has the first elected female AAOMS Trustee on the Board, and 3 of 6

Number of Full-Time and Part-Time Dental School Faculty by Gender, Race and Ethnicity, 2018–19 Academic Year

Hover over a segment and/or click on the tabs to see more details

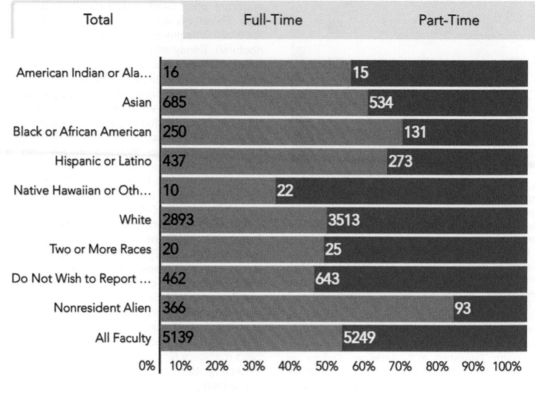

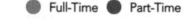

Fig. 8. ADEA first time enrollees by gender and race and full-time faculty 2019. (*From* ADEA Survey of Dental School Faculty, 2018-19, https://www.adea.org/data/Faculty/2018-2019-Survey. Copyright 2021 by the American Dental Education Association. Used with permission.)

District Caucus chairs are women. Members of URM will chair 6 AAOMS Committees and Special Committees for the year 2021 (AAOMS Today Jan/Feb 2021). The American Dental Association has had 4 female Presidents (1991, 2005, 2015, 2016), 1 Asian American (2002), 1 black (2009), and 2 Hispanics (2016 and 2022). There are more women and members of URM that are climbing the ranks for leadership in the demographic of dental leadership.

Dental school faculty totals 5139 for the 2018 to 2019 academic year, with white faculty at 2893, Asian, 685; Hispanic, 437; black, 25; American Indian/Native Hawaiian, 26 (2018-2019 Dental School Faculty in the United States ADEA Survey of Dental Schools). Looking at the ACS, women comprise 50% of medical graduates and now account for 40% of active residents in all surgical programs.[44] Presently, there are 82,000 members of the ACS: 15.9% are women, 9.7% are Fellows, and 39.3% of Resident Members are women, and there have been 3 female Presidents. The first AA member of the College was in 1913. In 2019, 2.6% of the nation's doctors and 7.3% of students enrolled in medical school identified as black or AA. Of 15,671 US medical school surgical faculty, 123 (0.79%) were AA women surgeons, with only 11 (0.54%) being tenured.

The need to increase diversity in health care and in the surgical and surgical subspecialty areas is compelling.[13,24,33,42,45–47] In 2004, the Institutes of Medicine (IOM) looked at and addressed the urgency of enhancing diversity, as the US demographics were shifting. The IOM report stated that more diverse health care providers would

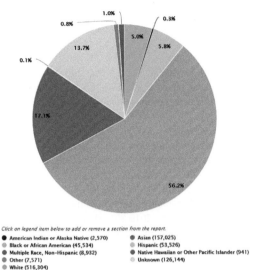

Click on legend item below to add or remove a section from the report.

- American Indian or Alaska Native (2,570)
- Asian (157,025)
- Black or African American (45,534)
- Hispanic (53,526)
- Multiple Race, Non–Hispanic (8,932)
- Native Hawaiian or Other Pacific Islander (941)
- Other (7,571)
- Unknown (126,144)
- White (516,304)

Fig. 9. Percentage of active physicians pie chart number and percentage of all active physicians by race/ethnicity, 2018. (*From* Diversity in Medicine: Facts and Figures 2019. Copyright © 1995-2020 Association of American Medical Colleges; Used with permission.)

lead to improved access to care for minorities and permit better communication and greater patient-centered care, as cultural competence is enhanced (https://www.nap.edu/caralog/10885/in-the-nations-compelling-interest-ensuring-

diversity-in-the-health Ensuring Diversity in the Health Care Workforce 2004). Workforce diversity continues to be an elusive goal at the highest levels of leadership, in Surgical Associations education, both medical and dental undergraduate schools and the faculty contingent, and dental/medical advanced education residencies. Lack of workforce diversity has been shown to have negative effects on patient outcomes, access to care, patient trust, employee retention, and workplace experiences. Race and sex concordance between patients and physicians has been associated with higher patient satisfaction for female and minority patients[48] and may help mitigate health care disparities affecting minority patients. Barriers to achieving balance for women and URM in the surgical and surgical subspecialty arenas include interview protocols and lack of interviewer bias training.[19,20,23,24,40,49–50] Other barriers include underwhelming recruitment strategies for URM/women; dearth of mentorship and sponsorship activities for less diverse student/resident groups; and minimal strategies to cultivate, nurture, and support advancement in the clinical/academic/leadership ladder for these groups.[51] Further exploration of the application and acceptance rates of students/trainees, along with academic faculty/workforce review, will allow expansion of opportunities for these groups and will be mandated in the future.

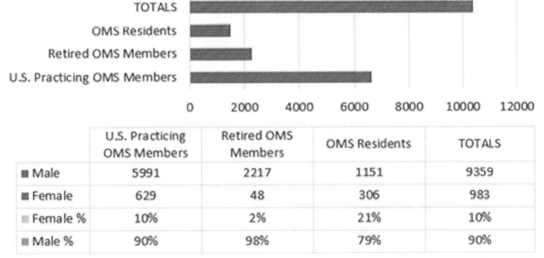

	U.S. Practicing OMS Members	Retired OMS Members	OMS Residents	TOTALS
Male	5991	2217	1151	9359
Female	629	48	306	983
Female %	10%	2%	21%	10%
Male %	90%	98%	79%	90%

Fig. 10. AAOMS membership and governance. AAOMS membership-gender comparison received May 18, 2021 from AAOMS headquarters. (*From* AAOMS Membership-Gender Comparison; used with permission of Dr. Wittich, the Exec. Dir for AAOMS.)

DISCLOSURE

B.L. Ferguson: Nothing to report. 100th President of American Association of Oral and Maxillofacial Surgeons (AAOMS) 2018. M. Morgan and S.B. Wilson: Neither have a commercial interest and have nothing to disclose.

REFERENCES

1. Truman Medical Center Archives.
2. Available at: https://www.trumed.org>about- us.
3. Peters G, University honors the first black woman to earn a medical degree from KU, KU Med Center News 08/24/2018.
4. Grutter v. Bollinger Supreme Court docket no. 02-241, citation 539 U.S. 306 (2003). Accessed May 18, 2021.
5. Aziz, H, Ducoin, C, Welch, D, et al, 2018 ACS governors survey: gender inequality and harassment remain a challenge in surgery bulletin. Bulletin of the American College of Surgeons. facs.facs.org/2-19/09/2019/2018-acs.
6. deCosta J, Xu J, Benentousi Z, et al. Women in surgery: challenges and opportunities. Int J Surg Glob Health 2018;1:e02.
7. West M, Hwang S, Maier R, et al. Ensuing equity, diversity and inclusion in academic surgery. Ann Surg 2018;268(3):403–7.
8. Sullivan L, Mittman I. The state of diversity in health professionals a century after Flexner. Acad Med 2010;85(2):246–53.
9. Flexner Report (Carnegie Foundation Bulletin Number Four). Available at: https://www.worldcat.org/oclc/9795002. Accessed on May 18, 2021.
10. Byrd WM, Clayton LA. An American Health Dilemma: race, medicine and health care in the US. New York: Rutledge; 2000.
11. Jones-Wilson F, Asbury C, Anderson DR, 1996 Encyclopedia of African American education ISBN 978-0-313-28931-6.
12. Aibana O, Swails J, Flores R, et al. Bridging the gap: holistic review to increase diversity in graduate medical education. Acad Med 2019;94(8):1137–41.
13. Silver JK, Bean AC, Slocum C, et al. Physician workforce disparities and patient care: a narrative review. Health Equity 2019;3(1):360–77.
14. Ali AM, McVay CL. Women in surgery: a history of adversity, resilience, and accomplishment. J Am Coll Surg 2016;223(4):670–3.
15. Wirtzfeld DA. The history of women in surgery. Can J Surg 2009;52(4): 317-20.
16. Hine DC. The corporeal and ocular veil: Dr Matilda A. Evans (1872-1935) and the complexity of southern history. J of Southern History 2004;70(1):3-34.
17. Changing the Face of Medicine. Available at: Cfmendicine.nim.nih.gov/physicians.biography_46. Accessed May 11, 2021.
18. Monarrez T, Washington K. Racial and ethnic representation in postsecondary education June 2020.
19. Koka S, Phasuk K, Kattadiyil MT, et al. Leadership diversity in dentistry: progress and lack thereof. J Am Dent Assoc 2021;152(2):85–8.
20. Weintraub K, Juliann Bluitt-Foster: trailblazers in dentistry, The New York Times, ISSN 0362-4331.
21. U.S. Census.gov, July 1, 2019.
22. ADEA first time enrollers by gender and race and full time faculty 2019. American Dental Educators Association. ADEA.org/snapshot(annual).
23. Lett LA, Murdock HM, Orji WU, et al. Trends in racial/ethnic representation among US medical students. JAMA Netw Open 2019;2(9):e1910490.
24. Baugh A, Baugh RF. Assessment of diversity outcomes in American medical school admissions: applying the Grutter legitimacy principles. Sustainability 2020;12(12):5211.
25. ACGME Surgical Residency Programs and Fellowship 2008 – 2018. Physician Specialty report of the ACGME and Association of American Medical Colleges.
26. AAMC Table 1.3 number and percentage of active physicians by sex and specialty. 2019. Available at: aamc.org/data-reports/workforce/interactive-data. Accessed April 18, 2021.
27. Burke AB, Cheng KL, Han JT, et al. Is gender associated with success in academic oral and maxillofacial surgery? J Oral Maxillofac Surg 2019;77(2):240–6.
28. Kolokythas A, Miloro M. Why do women choose to enter academic oral and maxillofacial surgery? J Oral Maxillofac Surg 2016;74(5):881–8.
29. Lopez EM, Farzal Z, Ebert CS Jr, et al. Recent trends in female and racial/ethnic minority groups in U.S. otolaryngology residency programs. Laryngoscope 2021;131(2):277–81.
30. AAMC Table 2.2 number and percentage of ACGME residents and fellows by sex and specialty. 2019. Available at. aamc.org/data-reports/interactive-data/acgme. Accessed April 18, 2021.
31. Michas F. Number of physicians in the U.S. by specialty and gender, 2019. 2021. Available at: statista.com/statics/439728/Feb 3. Accessed May 18, 2021.
32. Benay CE, Burneikis TA, Bobanga ID, et al. Academic Surgery, Leadership, and Diversity: Modern Workforce Analysis. Scientific Forum Health Services Research 2018;227(4 Supplement 2): E29.
33. Marino I, American AAOMS Membership – Gender Comparison Association of Oral and Maxillofacial Surgery Members.
34. Criddle TR, Gordon NC, Blakey G, et al. African Americans in oral and maxillofacial surgery: factors affecting career choice, satisfaction, and practice

patterns. J Oral Maxillofac Surg 2017;75(12): 2489–96.

5. Simon L, Candamo F, He P, et al. Gender differences in academic productivity and advancement among dental school faculty. J Womens Health (Larchmt) 2019;28(10):1350–4.

6. Sayre K, Carver KZ, Anderson S, et al. Barriers to women in oral and maxillofacial surgery: a cross sectional survey. J Oral Maxillofac Surg 2019; 77(9):e53.

7. Nieblas-Bedolla E, Williams JR, Christophers B, et al. Trends in race/ethnicity among applicants and matriculants to US surgical specialties, 2010-2018. JAMA Netw Open 2020;3(11):e2023509.

8. Choinski K, Lipsitz E, Indes J, et al. Trends in sex and racial/ethnic diversity in applicants to surgery residency and fellowship programs. JAMA Surg 2020;155(8):778–81.

9. Aspan M. Black women account for less than 3% of U.S. doctors. Is health care finally ready to face racism and sexism. 2020. Available at: Fortune.com. Accessed May 18, 2021.

0. AAMC Holistic Review in Medical School Admissions Students-Residents.aamc.org/2021.

1. Laskin DM. The role of women in academic oral and maxillofacial surgery. J Oral Maxillofac Surg 2015; 73(4):579.

2. Bruce AN, Battista A, Plankey MW, et al. Perceptions of gender-based discrimination during surgical training and practice. Med Educ Online 2015;20:25923.

3. Wallis CJD, Ravi B, Coburn N, et al. Comparison of postoperative outcomes among patients treated by male and female surgeons: a population based matched cohort study. BMJ 2017;359:j4366.https://doi.org/10.1136/bmj.j4366.

44. Accreditation Council for Graduate Medical Education. Data Resource Book Academic Year 2016–2017. www.acgme.org/About-Us/Publicans-and-Resources/Graduate-Medical-Education-Data-Resource Book.

45. Freischlag JA, Silva MM. Bouncing up: resilience and women in academic medicine. J Am Coll Surg 2016;223(2):215–20.

46. Atlas M. Female surgeons: how to thrive in a male dominated field. Available at: WWW.surgimate.com/blog 12/19/2019. Accessed May 11, 2021.

47. Marbin J, Rosenbluth G, Brim R, et al. Improving diversity in pediatric residency selection: using an equity framework to implement holistic review. J Grad Med Educ 2021;13(2):195–200.

48. Laveist TA, Nuru-Jeter A. Is doctor-patient race concordance associated with greater satisfaction with care? J Health Soc Behav 2002;43:296–306.

49. Valenzuela F, Romero Arenas MA. Underrepresented in surgery: (lack of) diversity in academic surgery faculty. J Surg Res 2020;254:170–4.

50. Hupp JR. Holistic review in residency admissions. J Oral Maxillofac Surg 2020;78(8):1217–8.

51. Yuce TK, Turner PL, Glass C, et al. National evaluation of racial/ethnic discrimination in US surgical residency programs. JAMA Surg 2020;155(6):526–8.

The Diversity Bonus in Oral and Maxillofacial Surgery

Catherine Haviland, DDS[a], Justine Sherylyn Moe, MD, DDS[b],*

KEYWORDS

- Health disparity • Diversity • Diversity bonus • Race • Gender • Underrepresented minority
- Health access

KEY POINTS

- The health care industry, surgical specialties, and OMS in particular are not reflective of the diverse makeup of the nation.
- For teams completing complex predictive, creative, and problem-solving tasks, such as OMS, there is no tradeoff between diversity and excellence. Rather, diversity provides a bonus.
- To achieve a diversity bonus diverse teams must learn to function effectively. Institutions must change policies related to admissions, hiring, and recruitment and invest in team communication and implicit bias training.
- A diversity bonus in OMS could potentially result in: expanded access to care, more equitable research, and attracting the best and brightest to the specialty.

INTRODUCTION
The State of Diversity

The US Census Bureau projects that by 2044 more than half of all Americans will belong to a minority group, with this value currently falling at around 40% of the population.[1,2] Yet the diversity of the nation is not reflected in the makeup of the health care industry. As with other surgical fields, oral and maxillofacial surgery (OMS) remains predominately White and male. It is therefore useful to consider the current state of racial and gender diversity within the specialty before considering how expanding diversity can enhance the profession.

Although half of all dental students were female in 2018, women fill only 16% of OMS residency positions and comprise only 8% of American Association of Oral and Maxillofacial Surgery memberships.[1] The same year, minority OMS residents made up only 32% of the total and 58% of this group were Asian.[3] Faculty positions within OMS, medical, and dental schools follow a similar distribution of White male predominance.[1] Women generally make up only 40% full-time faculty and fill only 20% of chair and program director positions.[1] Major OMS governing bodies suffer from even more severely limited representation.[1] As an illustration, all of the officers and trustees of the American Association of Oral and Maxillofacial Surgery for 2020 were White and only one was female.[4] Based on these metrics, OMS currently lacks representation from women and predominately Black and Hispanic underrepresented minorities.[1]

The profession is not representative of the racial and gendered makeup of the population at large. One might appropriately query why exactly this is problematic. Generally, the argument is a moral one. Yet in a capitalist society driven by financial gain, normative arguments usually fall short of producing tangible results.[5] Maintenance of the status quo and pushback against diversity initiatives generally stem from an inherent belief that there is a tradeoff between diversity and excellence.[5]

The authors have no disclosures.
[a] University of Michigan, Med Inn Building, 1500 East Medical Center Drive, SPC 5827, Ann Arbor, MI 48109-5827, USA; [b] University of Michigan, Med Inn Building, Floor 2 Room C213, 1500 East Medical Center Drive, SPC 5827, Ann Arbor, MI 48109-5827, USA
* Corresponding author.
E-mail address: jusmoe@med.umich.edu

Oral Maxillofacial Surg Clin N Am 33 (2021) 505–513
https://doi.org/10.1016/j.coms.2021.05.008
1042-3699/21/© 2021 Elsevier Inc. All rights reserved.

For example, a university may fear that selecting applicants to expand diversity will reduce its academic prowess. The diversity bonus theorem, as proposed by Scott Page, provides a mathematical basis for undermining this false assumption.[5] It postulates that in specific environments, diversity is an absolute necessity to creating the most successful team. There is no tradeoff.

Although the following discussion describes the benefits of diverse teams, it is worth bearing in mind that discussions of diversity tend to emphasize proof of purpose. To change the status quo, it seems necessary to outline the moral and financial gains that diversity can bring to an organization. For those who are a part of the majority group, however, there is never a need to provide proof of utility in places of power.[6] The status quo is a given, whereas diversity is often perceived as something in which one can choose to partake. The theorem provides an incentive for needed change while acknowledging that its existence is inherently discriminatory.

DEFINITIONS
Categories of Diversity

To best understand the diversity bonus, one must first consider the definition of diversity itself. Diversity necessitates the existence of a group. An individual is not inherently diverse but rather brings diversity to the group because they differ from the other members in some way.[5] What is diverse in one team may not be in another. Another useful framework for the proceeding discussion involves the division of diversity into two broad categories: identity diversity and cognitive diversity. Identity diversity consists of categorical differences, such as race, gender, and sexual orientation.[5] Alternatively, cognitive diversity describes subtle variations in the way one thinks, which is influenced by membership in an identity group.[5]

When unpacking identity diversity, it is useful to consider three representative and interrelated models: (1) the iceberg, (2) the timber-framed house, and (3) the cloud. The iceberg model postulates that there are identity traits visible to the rest of the world, such as skin color or age, which represent the tip of the iceberg, with a host of invisible factors, such as religion, sexual orientation, and culture, lying below the water level.[5] When seeking out diversity, it is easy to erroneously make inferences about these invisible factors based on what is visible. Page recounts the tale of a Japanese American who was hired to manage a company's Asian American client list. He quit the position on discovering that the company had failed to consider the base of the iceberg. The client list was composed of entirely Korean Americans.[5]

The timber-framed house model shows that identities are interconnected and separating the impact of individual identity traits is problematic.[5] When one component is removed, the whole house may crumble. This framework describes the concept of intersectionality, or the complex and numerous discriminations and disadvantages of a person or group because of overlapping identities and experiences. The consideration of race and gender separately, for example, can overlook complex forms of oppression and lead to bias.[7] Take for example, that 3.6% of full-time medical faculty positions in 2018 were held by Black individuals.[8] Yet nearly 60% of these positions were held by Black women. Intersectionality considers that there is an even greater disparity of Black male medical faculty than would be exposed by considering race or gender in isolation.

The cloud model offers a final useful framework for considering the pitfalls of categorizing groups based on identity diversity. Within individual identity categories (eg, Asian female physicians) are a heterogenous set of people with a diverse cognitive repertoire (eg, subspecialty, career focus, political view, social class, skin color, family structure). Identity categories should be thought of as neighboring and overlapping clouds.[5] For example, a group consisting of male neurosurgeons older than the age of 40 might include such disparate figures as Ben Carson, Sanjay Gupta, and Christopher Duntsch; selecting one of these individuals as a representative to provide perspective for the entire group would be impossible because the group itself is so diverse. The cloud model serves as a reminder to avoid token examples of representation, because one individual cannot represent an entire category of people.

All of these identity factors in turn contribute to cognitive diversity. Life experience influences the way in which one views the world, their knowledge base, and their approach to problem solving. When workers are problem solving and thinking creatively, they perform better when identity diversity is present and can solve issues that have perplexed experts.[9,10]

Professions driven by consumer interaction, such as medicine and OMS, are thus best served by embracing identity differences. Individuals from different backgrounds and life experiences are needed to anticipate and understand the needs of their patients and communities they serve. For example, in many Hispanic communities bottled water is preferred over tap water because of historically negative experiences with water quality.[11] A provider without knowledge of his preference or its origins is poorly fit to design a ublic health campaign to improve fluoridation mong Hispanic and Latino communities. The roblems that we choose to address and the issues we value depend on our identity and personal xperiences. An individual who has never used a wheelchair is less likely to consider physical ccessibility when designing an office space.[5]

Identity diversity additionally prompts the recognition that cognitive diversity exists.[6] The presence f someone with a different identity changes the ehavior of other group members. Identity diverse roups are more tolerant of disagreements ecause they expect these disagreements to rise.[6,12] There is an inherent expectation that nose who look like you will share your beliefs. dentity diversity disrupts this assumption.[6,13] For xample, White jurors in diverse groups identified nore missing evidence, had fewer inaccuracies, were more willing to discuss race as a factor in egal decisions, and raised more novel ideas than lid White jurors in nondiverse groups.[14] The nere presence of identity diversity triggers recognition that cognitive diversity is present and valuable.

Categories of Work

To apply these definitions to forms of teamwork, we must consider four distinct categories of work: (1) cognitive work involves use of the mind, (2) physical work involves use of the hands, (3) outine work is managed by machines, and (4) nonroutine work requires human cognition.[5] Diversity bonuses are not achievable in all categories and some professions are more readily able to achieve a bonus than others. Physical work and outine work are less likely to benefit from diversity. For example, the best assembly line worker completing physical routine tasks is the one with the most speed and efficiency, and the best group ncludes workers with similar, rather than varied, characteristics.

Alternatively, cognitive nonroutine professions, such as law, politics, and OMS, which dominate he modern economy, are uniquely able to achieve a diversity bonus.[5] Such professions require a eam effort for success because they have many dimensions, require sharing of information, and he complex tasks they complete cannot be decomposed into individual parts.[5] When managing a complex facial trauma case, for example, multidisciplinary collaboration between individuals with expertise in maxillofacial reconstruction, maxillofacial prosthodontics, anesthesiology, speech and language pathology, physical therapy, and nutrition, may be needed to optimize the patient outcome. From a research perspective, 80% of the top 200 most cited OMS papers are collaborations of two or more individuals, which suggests that diverse backgrounds and viewpoints leads to impactful research.[15]

The Diversity Theorem

The diversity theorem describes how bonuses are obtained on predictive, creative, and problem-solving tasks. To understand the theorem broadly, an ideal stock portfolio can be considered, in which a diverse portfolio generally performs better than one that relies on only a few stocks.[5] Furthermore, diverse teams need not accept what is average. Rather, a diverse team is equivalent to a portfolio where stocks, or in our case ideas, which perform poorly can be dropped. The team achieves a bonus by selecting the best idea from a diverse set.

Predictive Tasks

Predictive tasks are defined as determining the outcome of an intervention, such as treatment of a patient.[5] The accuracy of a group prediction in such a setting can be mathematically modeled. The diversity prediction theorem states that collective error = average error − predictive diversity (**Fig. 1**).[5] Prediction error refers to the square of the difference between the true value and the prediction.[5] Collective error is the prediction error of the average of the group members' predictions. The average error is the average of the group members' prediction errors. Predictive diversity is the variance of the group members' predictions.

To better understand the theorem, it is useful to consider a simple numerical example. Consider a group of three students guessing the number of gumballs in a jar where the correct answer is 50. The groups guesses are 25, 75, and 100. The average prediction of the group is therefore 67. When using these values in the theorem, CE

Diversity Prediction Theorem

Collective error (CE) = average error (AE) -predictive diversity (PD)

Group ability = average ability + diversity

TV = true value

$$CE = \left[\left(\frac{Prediction\ A + Prediction\ B + Prediction\ C...}{Total\ \#\ of\ predictions}\right) - TV\right]^2$$

$$AE = \frac{(TV - Prediction\ A)^2 + (TV - Prediction\ B)^2 + (TV - Prediction\ C)^2}{Total\ \#\ of\ predictions}$$

PD = Variance of predictions

Fig. 1. Diversity bonus theorem. (*Adapted from* Page SE. The Diversity Bonus: How Great Teams Pay Off in the Knowledge Economy. Princeton University Press; 2019.)

(278) = AE (1250) – PD (972).[5] The collective error of the group is much smaller than the average error because the group's predictions were diverse (**Fig. 2**).

A further extension of this logic is that group ability = average ability + diversity.[5] It follows that a group's ability depends on diversity and average ability to equal extent. Diverse groups are more accurate than the average of their members.[5] When considering whether to add a team member, the not half bad rule comes into play. As long as the individual is no more than 50% less accurate than the other group members, they will improve the groups accuracy by bringing diversity. This explains why predictions about weather or climate change average numerous diverse models to create the most accurate one.[5] Ultimately the theorem demonstrates that when considering predictive tasks, there is no tradeoff between ability and diversity, and both make an equal contribution.[5]

Creative Tasks

When considering creative tasks or the generation of new ideas, the diversity bonus also comes into play. As an example, one might consider a team generating a novel surgical approach.

Assuming each individual brings a certain number of novel ideas, the most successful team in this scenario is not necessarily composed of the most individually creative people. The most creative team incorporates individuals with nonoverlapping ideas. Perhaps Person A and B both have five novel approaches but three of them are shared by both (**Fig. 3**). Less creative person C may have only three novel approaches but if these approaches are unique she generates a more creative team when paired with person A or B (eight novel ideas) than when A and B are paired together (seven novel ideas). Therefore, when forming groups, the number of outside the box ideas an individual can contribute matters more than the total

$$CE = \left[\left(\frac{25+75+100}{3}\right) - 50\right]^2 = 278$$

$$AE = \frac{(50-25)^2+(75-50)^2+(100-50)^2}{3} = 1250$$

$$PD = 972$$

$$278 = 1250 - 972$$

Fig. 2. Numerical example of the theorem. (*Adapted from* Page SE. The Diversity Bonus: How Great Teams Pay Off in the Knowledge Economy. Princeton University Press; 2019.)

number of ideas they possess.[5] Moreover, sharing ideas within groups further compounds creativity through superadditivity.[5] In our case, Person A with five novel ideas could form 10 unique pairs, the grouping of Person A and Person B could form 21 unique pairs, whereas the grouping of Person A or B with Person C could form 28 unique pairs (**Fig. 4**).[5]

Problem-Solving Tasks

Problem-solving tasks are understood as those tasks that involve generation of solutions that meet particular criteria or that make improvements to what already exists.[5] Individuals have a set of tools at their disposal to solve problems, and possess a certain level of mastery with each tool. Mathematically, the probability that an individual solves a problem with a specific tool is the product of the individual's mastery of that tool and the specific tool's potential.[5]

In certain disciplines, tools must be learned in a specific order; one cannot acquire the next tool before learning the first. In these situations, diversity bonuses are not possible. Alternatively, in such fields as surgery, an individual might acquire a range of tools in any order. For example, a surgeon proficient with microvascular surgery need not be an expert on implant placement first.

The best problem-solving group consists of the highest facility individuals with each tool. This does not imply that the group is composed of the individuals with the greatest ability across all tools.[5] Consider a team of two oral surgeons where each surgeon's mastery with tools, such as implant placement, temporomandibular joint procedures, and orthognathic surgery, is either 60% or 80% (**Fig. 5**). Assume each of these tools has a 50% chance of solving the problem at hand. The team composed of the two highest-ability surgeons, Person A and B, will not perform as well as a more diverse team with lower ability individuals. When the number of tools available expands beyond what any single individual could master, selection based on diversity rather than ability alone delivers a bonus.[5]

DISCUSSION
Diversity Improves Access to Care

Disparities in access to care are pervasive throughout the health care industry and present one of the major challenges currently facing global health. Within OMS, minority communities are more likely to face reduced access and quality of care, and have poorer treatment outcomes. Non-White, low-income, and physically disabled individuals are more likely to require oral surgical

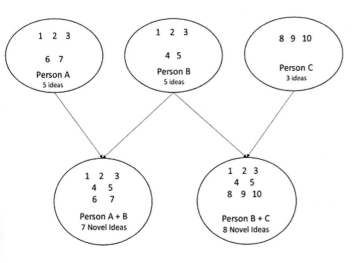

Fig. 3. The most creative team is not composed of the most creative people. (*Adapted from* Page SE. The Diversity Bonus: How Great Teams Pay Off in the Knowledge Economy. Princeton University Press; 2019.)

care.[16] Regarding oral cancer, Black race is associated with more advanced stage at diagnosis and poorer survival after adjusting for other factors.[17] When implemented effectively, expanding diversity of practitioners can result in enhanced access to care for those in underserved communities.

There are numerous studies demonstrating that minority dentists and physicians provide more care to minority patients and those who are underserved, uninsured, and Medicaid recipients.[18–22] Minority race of the provider is the strongest predictor of serving the underserved.[19] This phenomenon seems to be caused by a combination of patient preference and practice location. Patients are more likely to prefer a race-concordant provider if they hold a belief of racial discrimination within the health care industry.[23] Diversity of providers additionally enhances communication and satisfaction of care for patients.[24,25] From a location standpoint, Black and Hispanic students in medicine and dentistry report a greater intent to practice in underserved and urban environments than their White or Asian counterparts **(Fig. 6)**.[26,27] On an anecdotal note, Dr Aziz relays in his 2010 piece on diversity his own experience treating a higher proportion of Muslim patients than other surgeons and as a result becoming an expert on oral submucous fibrosis, which is

$$\frac{\text{\# unique ideas} \times \text{\# of ideas each idea can be paired with}}{2}$$

For example: $(8 \times 7)/2 = 28$. The first idea of the 8 can form 7 pairs.

Fig. 4. Mathematical basis of superadditivity. (*Adapted from* Page SE. The Diversity Bonus: How Great Teams Pay Off in the Knowledge Economy. Princeton University Press; 2019.)

prevalent in patients from the Indian subcontinent.[17] This is not to imply, however, that minority students should be admitted with the expectation of practicing in underserved communities; rather, expanding access to care is a natural by-product of increasing diversity.

Moreover, training in a diverse environment enhances the educational experience of all students and increases the likelihood they will go on to treat diverse communities.[18] Perception of diversity within dental school and inclusion of diversity content within the curriculum is positively correlated with the perceived ability to work with diverse populations.[28] Learning among a diverse group improves learning outcomes, understanding differences, active thinking, and intellectual engagement.[18]

Research Bias

Medical research has a long discriminatory history and contributes to the perpetuation of health care disparities. Subjects selected for clinical research are disproportionately White and male. Some data report values of 5% of clinical trial participants are Black and 1% Hispanic.[29] Historical disparities in gendered involvement have led to negative outcomes, such as increased rates of adverse drug reactions in women.[29,30] Most evidence-based medicine is thus not applicable to most of the population. Continuing disparities in research are multifactorial and include poor communication, access barriers, language barriers, and a historical mistrust among minorities of the medical infrastructure.[31,32] The Tuskegee study and forced sterilization are a few of the more well-known abuses of the medical system on the most vulnerable.[31] It is unsurprising then that minority research participants report being

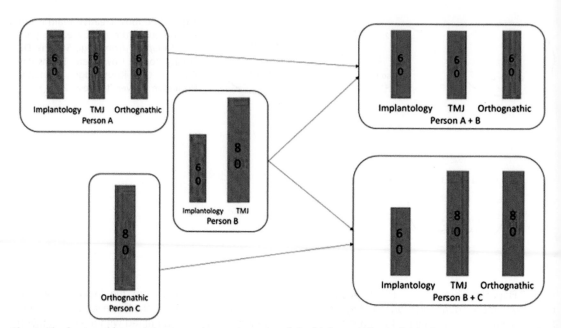

Fig. 5. The best problem-solving team does not consist of the highest-ability individuals. TMJ, temporomandibular joint. (*Adapted from* Page SE. The Diversity Bonus: How Great Teams Pay Off in the Knowledge Economy. Princeton University Press; 2019.)

more willing to join a project if one of the researchers is also a minority individual.[29,32]

Within the realm of OMS, cephalometric analysis and normal values are primarily based on the facial norms of White patients.[17] Yet around a third of those who receive orthognathic treatment are non-White.[33] Soft tissue and cephalometric norms have been shown to vary widely across various ethnic and racial groups.[34–36] Perception of an esthetic facial profile is moreover influenced by such factors as culture, socioeconomic status, education, and gender.[37,38] Understanding the esthetics and cultural preferences of diverse patients is necessary to provide the best care.[17,34] Expanding diversity of the profession may encourage minority participation in research, generate researchers more likely to take race into consideration, and ensure greater cultural understanding of diverse research participants.[32]

Capturing the Diversity Bonus: Implications for Practice

To successfully capture the diversity bonus, the OMS specialty needs to adopt a paradigm shift on the importance and advantage of diversity within OMS and among team members. Assessments of team culture, discrimination, harassment, and implicit bias, and policy changes relating to recruitment and retention need to be prioritized. Barriers and challenges for

underrepresented minorities in OMS need to be identified and addressed. Multiple strategies to improve team diversity have been previously described as follows:

- Formation of a diversity mission statement and leadership positions
- Community engagement for recruitment[39]
- Changes in admissions practices
  - ○ Limit overreliance on examination scores, which have historically been lower for

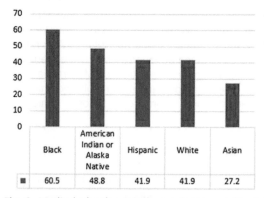

Fig. 6. Medical school matriculants intent to practice in underserved areas. (*Data from* Diversity in Medicine: Facts and Figures 2019. Available at: https://www.aamc.org/data-reports/workforce/report/diversity-medicine-facts-and-figures-2019. Accessed December 28, 2020.)

underrepresented minorities and often fail to correlate with clinical performance.[25,40] Consider such factors as personal challenges or creativity at solving practice cases.

- Dedicated committee on minority enrollment. Race-neutral admissions practices result in a 70% drop in underrepresented minority students.[41]
- Changes in hiring practices
  - Advertise positions broadly and limit reliance on personal networks when selecting interviewees for faculty positions.[42]
  - Implement the Rooney Rule, which has been successful in the sports realm. For each position one female or underrepresented minority should be interviewed.[43,44]
- Create a more welcoming and civil workplace environment and workplace culture
  - Mandatory training on implicit bias, sexual harassment, cultural competence, and social norms approach to address reports from female, minority, and other diverse groups of bias, harassment, and limited knowledge of resources available to address concerns when they arise.[45–47]
- Provide support throughout training
  - Team communication: use of validated systems, such as the Oxford NOTECHS tool, to improve and evaluate diverse team performance while in the operating room.[48]
- Objective assessments of the impact of policy changes

It should be noted that the development of policies to create diverse teams without a comprehensive assessment of systemic barriers to diversity have not been shown to actualize long-term gains, and can create additional challenges, including tokenism, conflict, and reduced communication into team environments.[49] A veritable culture change and multipronged approach to creating diverse teams in OMS are necessary to capture the diversity bonus.

The Talent Pool

To ensure its future success the OMS profession must attract the best and brightest minds to the specialty.[50] In a country that is half female, majority minority, and religiously and culturally diverse, if certain groups are excluded, either willfully or because they do not feel welcomed, the profession will suffer.[5] Practitioners must understand the needs, causes of disease burden, and best suited solutions for increasingly diverse communities.[39,51]

SUMMARY

The diversity bonus theorem postulates that in specific environments, diversity is an absolute necessity to creating the most successful team. The theorem dispels the myth that institutions must choose between diversity and excellence. Within OMS this bonus is captured in numerous ways, including through expanded access to care, more equitable and relevant research, and attracting the best and brightest to the specialty. To capture this bonus the profession must invest in policy changes to admissions and hiring and offer training in communication, cultural competency, and implicit bias.

CLINICS CARE POINTS

The diversity bonus theorem leads to several practically useful adages.

- The losing side bonus: In group decision-making (eg, surgical decisions, academic committees), in order for the group to be useful, an individual must, before being swayed by group discussion, be on the losing side of some votes. If an individual were always on the winning side, they would make equally accurate decisions without being part of a group.[5] The group thus makes a more accurate decision than the individual only when the individual is sometimes on the losing side.

- The meritocratic fallacy: The best team is not made of the traditionally best individuals but rather the best and most diverse individuals.[5]

- The not half bad rule: On predictive tasks, an individual should be selected for a group if they are not more than 50% less accurate than the other group members.[5]

- No test rule: No single objective measure, such as a test score, can be used to form the most creative group because an individuals' creative contribution is dependent on the new ideas they can offer to an existing group.[5] A new idea in one group setting may not be novel in another because what constitutes a new idea depends on what ideas the group already possesses.

- Knowledge integration: For tasks that require integration of knowledge, such as the development of a treatment plan for a patient with head and neck cancers that will result in the best outcomes and least complications, each individual's knowledge can help to eliminate options and arrive at a final decision.[5]

REFERENCES

1. Lee JS, Aziz SR. Diversity and cultural competency in oral and maxillofacial surgery. Oral Maxillofac Surg Clin North Am 2020;32(3):389–405.

2. United States Census Bureau. US census bureau quick facts: United States. Available at: https://www-census-gov.proxy.lib.umich.edu/quickfacts/fact/table/US/PST045218. Accessed December 28, 2020.

3. American Dental Association. Enrollment in advanced dental education programs by gender and race/ethnicity, 2018-19. Available at: https://www-ada-org.proxy.lib.umich.edu/en/~/media/ADA/Science%20and%20Research/HPI/Files/SADV_2018-19. Accessed December 28 2020.

4. American Association of Oral and Maxillofacial Surgery. 2019-2020 AAOMS officers and trustees. Available at: https://www.aaoms.org/about/board-of-trustees. Accessed, December 28, 2020.

5. Page SE. The diversity bonus. Princeton: Princeton University Press; 2019.

6. Phillips KW. What is the real value of diversity in organizations? Questioning our assumptions. In: Page SE, editor. The diversity bonus. Princeton: Princeton University Press; 2019. p. P223–47.

7. Cole ER. Intersectionality and research in psychology. Am Psychol 2009;64(3):170–80.

8. Association of American Medical Colleges. US medical school faculty by sex and race/ethnicity. Available at: https://www.aamc.org/system/files/reports/1/18table8.pdf. Accessed December 28, 2020.

9. Sparber C. Racial diversity and aggregate productivity in U.S. industries: 1980-2000. South Econ J 2009;75:829–56.

10. Lakhani KR, Jeppesen LB. Getting unusual suspects to solve R&D puzzles. In: Harvard Business review. Available at. hbr.org/2007/05/getting-unusual-suspects-to-solve-rd-puzzles. Accessed December 28, 2020.

11. Scherzer T, Barker JC, Pollick H, et al. Water consumption beliefs and practices in a rural Latino community: implications for fluoridation. J Public Health Dent 2010;70(4):337–43.

12. Phillips KW. The effects of categorically based expectations on minority influence: the importance of congruence. Pers Soc Psychol Bull 2003;29(1):3–13.

13. Phillips KW, Loyd Denise L. When surface and deep-level diversity collide: the effects on dissenting group members. Organ Behav Hum Decis Process 2006;99(2):143–60.

14. Sommers SR. On racial diversity and group decision making. J Pers Soc Psychol 2006;90(4):597–612.

15. Aslam-Pervez N, Lubek J. Most cited publications in oral and maxillofacial surgery: a bibliometric analysis. Oral Maxillofac Surg 2018;22(1):25–37.

16. Moeller JF, Chen H, Manski RJ. Diversity in the use of specialized dental services by older adults in the United States. J Public Health Dent 2019;79(2):160–74.

17. Shiboski CH, Schmidt BL, Jordan RC. Racial disparity in stage at diagnosis and survival among adults with oral cancer in the US. Community Dent Oral Epidemiol 2007;35(3):233–40.

18. Tedesco LA. Post-affirmative action Supreme Court decision: new challenges for academic institutions. J Dent Educ 2005;69:1212–21.

19. Saha S, Shipman SA. Race-neutral versus race-conscious workforce policy to improve access to care. Health Aff 2008;27(1):234–45.

20. Okunseri C, Bajorunaite R, Abena A, et al. Racial/ethnic disparities in the acceptance of Medicaid patients in dental practices. J Public Health Dent 2008;68(3):149–53.

21. Solomon ES, William CR, Sinkford JC. Practice location characteristics of black dentists in Texas. J Dent Educ 2001;65:571–4.

22. Komaromy M, Grumbach K, Drake M. The role of black and Hispanic physicians in providing health care for the underserved populations. N Engl J Med 1996;334:1305–10.

23. Chen FM, Fryer GE, Phillips RL, et al. Patients' beliefs about racism, preferences for physician race, and satisfaction with care. Ann Fam Med 2005;3(2):138–43.

24. Mitchell DA, Lassiter SL. Addressing health care disparities and increasing workforce diversity: the next step for the dental, medical, and public health professions. Am J Public Health 2006;96(12):2093–7.

25. Smith C, Ester TV, Inglehart MR. Providing care for underserved patients: the role of dental education. J Dent Educ 2005;69(1):112–3.

26. Diversity in medicine: facts and figures 2019. Available at: https://www.aamc.org/data-reports/workforce/report/diversity-medicine-facts-and-figures-2019. Accessed December 28, 2020.

27. Wanchek T, Cook BJ, Valachovic RW. Annual ADEA survey of dental school seniors: 2017 graduating class. J Dent Educ 2018;82:524–39.

28. Novak KF, Whitehead AW, Close JM, et al. Students' perceived importance of diversity exposure and training in dental education. J Dent Educ 2004;68:355–60.

29. The Society for Women's Health Research United States Food and Drug Administration Office of Women's Health. Dialogues on diversifying clinical trials: successful strategies for engaging women and minorities in clinical trials. 2011. Available at: https://www.fda.gov/downloads/ScienceResearch/Special Topics/WomensHealthResearch/UCM334959.pdf. Accessed December 28, 2020.

30. Zucker I, Prendergast BJ. Sex differences in pharmacokinetics predict adverse drug reactions in women. Biol Sex Diffe 2020;11:32.

31. George S, Duran N, Norris K. A systematic review of barriers and facilitators to minority research participation among African Americans, Latinos, Asian Americans, and Pacific Islanders. Am J Public Health 2014;104(2):16–31.

32. Branson RD, Davis K, Butker KL. African American participation in clinical research: importance, barriers, and solutions. Am J Surg 2007;193:32.

33. Venugoplan SR, Nanda V, Turkistani K, et al. Discharge patterns of orthognathic surgeries in the United States. J Oral Maxillofac Surg 2012;70(1):77–86.

34. Heir JS, Sandhu BS, Barber HD. Considerations for esthetic facial surgery in the African-American patient. Atlas Oral Maxillofac Surg Clin North Am 2000;8:113–25.

35. Khosravanifard B, Rakhshan V, Raeesi E. Factors influencing attractiveness of soft tissue profile. Oral Surg Oral Med Oral Pathol Oral Radiol 2013;115:29–37.

36. Shindoi JM, Matsumoto Y, Sato Y, et al. Soft tissue cephalometric norms for orthognathic and cosmetic surgery. J Oral Maxillofac Surg 2013;71(1):24–30.

37. Mousavi S, Mohammad S, Ghorani P, et al. Effects of laterality on esthetic preferences of orthodontists, maxillofacial surgeons, and laypeople regarding the lip position and facial convexity: a psychometric clinical trial. Oral Maxillofac Surg 2019;23(4):439–51.

38. Nomura M, Motegi E, Hatch JP, et al. Esthetic preferences of European American, Hispanic American, Japanese, and African judges for soft-tissue profiles. Am J Orthod Dentofacial Orthop 2009;135:S87–95.

39. Formicola AJ, Klyvert M, McIntosh J, et al. Creating an environment for diversity in dental schools: one school's approach. J Dent Educ 2003;67(5):491–9.

40. Ranney RR, Wilson MB, Bennett RB. Evaluation of applicants to predoctoral dental education programs: review of the literature. J Dent Educ 2005;69(10):1095–106.

41. Cohen JJ. The consequences of premature abandonment of affirmative action in medical school admissions. JAMA 2003;289:1143.

42. Shubeck SP, Newman EA, Vitous AC, et al. Hiring practices of US academic surgery departments: challenges and opportunities for more inclusive hiring. J Surg Res 2020;254:23–30.

43. Butler PD, Longaker MT, Britt LD. Addressing the paucity of underrepresented minorities in academic surgery: can the "Rooney Rule" be applied to academic surgery? Am J Surg 2010;199(2):255–62.

44. Dossett LA, Mulholland MW, Newman EA. Building high-performing teams in academic surgery: the opportunities and challenges of inclusive recruitment strategies. Acad Med 2019;94(8):1142–5.

45. Criddle TR, Gordon NC, Blakey G, et al. African Americans in oral and maxillofacial surgery: factors affecting career choice, satisfaction and practice patterns. J Oral Maxillofac Surg 2015;73(9):57.

46. Zurayk LF, Cheng KL, Zemplenyi M, et al. Perceptions of sexual harassment in oral and maxillofacial surgery training and practice. J Oral Maxillofac Surg 2019;77(12):2377–85.

47. Uppgaard R. Addressing gender discrimination in oral and maxillofacial surgery via the social norms approach. J Oral Maxillofac Surg 2018;76(8):1604–5.

48. Mishra A, Catchpole K, McCulloch P. The Oxford NOTECHS System: reliability and validity of a tool for measuring teamwork behaviour in the operating theatre. Qual Saf Health Care 2009;18:104–8.

49. Phillips K. How diversity works. Sci Am 2014;311(4):42–7.

50. Assael LA. The diversity imperative: essential to a specialty's success. J Oral Maxillofac Surg 2010;68(8):1709–10.

51. Hupp JR. Our diversity: celebrating a century of the AAOMS. J Oral Maxillofac Surg 2018;76(1):1–2.

UNITED STATES POSTAL SERVICE®
Statement of Ownership, Management, and Circulation
(All Periodicals Publications Except Requester Publications)

1. Publication Title	2. Publication Number	3. Filing Date
ORAL & MAXILLOFACIAL SURGERY CLINICS OF NORTH AMERICA	006 – 362	9/18/2021

4. Issue Frequency	5. Number of Issues Published Annually	6. Annual Subscription Price
FEB, MAY, AUG, NOV	4	$401.00

7. Complete Mailing Address of Known Office of Publication *(Not printer)* *(Street, city, county, state, and ZIP+4®)*

ELSEVIER INC.
230 Park Avenue, Suite 800
New York, NY 10169

Contact Person
Malathi Samayan

Telephone *(Include area code)*
91-44-4299-4507

8. Complete Mailing Address of Headquarters or General Business Office of Publisher *(Not printer)*

ELSEVIER INC.
230 Park Avenue, Suite 800
New York, NY 10169

9. Full Names and Complete Mailing Addresses of Publisher, Editor, and Managing Editor *(Do not leave blank)*

Publisher *(Name and complete mailing address)*

Dolores Meloni, ELSEVIER INC.
1600 JOHN F KENNEDY BLVD. SUITE 1800
PHILADELPHIA, PA 19103-2899

Editor *(Name and complete mailing address)*

JOHN VASSALLO, ELSEVIER INC.
1600 JOHN F KENNEDY BLVD. SUITE 1800
PHILADELPHIA, PA 19103-2899

Managing Editor *(Name and complete mailing address)*

PATRICK MANLEY, ELSEVIER INC.
1600 JOHN F KENNEDY BLVD. SUITE 1800
PHILADELPHIA, PA 19103-2899

10. Owner *(Do not leave blank. If the publication is owned by a corporation, give the name and address of the corporation immediately followed by the names and addresses of all stockholders owning or holding 1 percent or more of the total amount of stock. If not owned by a corporation, give the names and addresses of the individual owners. If owned by a partnership or other unincorporated firm, give its name and address as well as those of each individual owner. If the publication is published by a nonprofit organization, give its name and address.)*

Full Name	Complete Mailing Address
WHOLLY OWNED SUBSIDIARY OF REED/ELSEVIER, US HOLDINGS	1600 JOHN F KENNEDY BLVD. SUITE 1800 PHILADELPHIA, PA 19103-2899

11. Known Bondholders, Mortgagees, and Other Security Holders Owning or Holding 1 Percent or More of Total Amount of Bonds, Mortgages, or Other Securities. If none, check box ► ☐ None

Full Name	Complete Mailing Address
N/A	

12. Tax Status *(For completion by nonprofit organizations authorized to mail at nonprofit rates)* *(Check one)*
The purpose, function, and nonprofit status of this organization and the exempt status for federal income tax purposes:
☒ Has Not Changed During Preceding 12 Months
☐ Has Changed During Preceding 12 Months *(Publisher must submit explanation of change with this statement)*

PS Form **3526**, July 2014 *(Page 1 of 4 (see instructions page 4))* PSN: 7530-01-000-9931 PRIVACY NOTICE: See our privacy policy on www.usps.com

---

13. Publication Title	14. Issue Date for Circulation Data Below
ORAL & MAXILLOFACIAL SURGERY CLINICS OF NORTH AMERICA	MAY 2021

15. Extent and Nature of Circulation		Average No. Copies Each Issue During Preceding 12 Months	No. Copies of Single Issue Published Nearest to Filing Date
a. Total Number of Copies *(Net press run)*		620	546
b. Paid Circulation *(By Mail and Outside the Mail)*	(1) Mailed Outside-County Paid Subscriptions Stated on PS Form 3541 (Include paid distribution above nominal rate, advertiser's proof copies, and exchange copies)	487	449
	(2) Mailed In-County Paid Subscriptions Stated on PS Form 3541 (Include paid distribution above nominal rate, advertiser's proof copies, and exchange copies)	0	0
	(3) Paid Distribution Outside the Mails Including Sales Through Dealers and Carriers, Street Vendors, Counter Sales, and Other Paid Distribution Outside USPS®	74	57
	(4) Paid Distribution by Other Classes of Mail Through the USPS (e.g., First-Class Mail®)	0	0
c. Total Paid Distribution *(Sum of 15b (1), (2), (3), and (4))* ►		561	506
d. Free or Nominal Rate Distribution *(By Mail and Outside the Mail)*	(1) Free or Nominal Rate Outside-County Copies included on PS Form 3541	43	25
	(2) Free or Nominal Rate In-County Copies Included on PS Form 3541	0	0
	(3) Free or Nominal Rate Copies Mailed at Other Classes Through the USPS (e.g., First-Class Mail)	0	0
	(4) Free or Nominal Rate Distribution Outside the Mail (Carriers or other means)	43	25
e. Total Free or Nominal Rate Distribution *(Sum of 15d (1), (2), (3) and (4))* ►		43	25
f. Total Distribution *(Sum of 15c and 15e)* ►		604	531
g. Copies not Distributed *(See Instructions to Publishers #4 (page #3))* ►		16	15
h. Total *(Sum of 15f and g)* ►		620	546
i. Percent Paid *(15c divided by 15f times 100)* ►		92.88%	95.29%

If you are claiming electronic copies, go to line 16 on page 3. If you are not claiming electronic copies, skip to line 17 on page 3.

16. Electronic Copy Circulation		Average No. Copies Each Issue During Preceding 12 Months	No. Copies of Single Issue Published Nearest to Filing Date
a. Paid Electronic Copies	►		
b. Total Paid Print Copies (Line 15c) + Paid Electronic Copies (Line 16a)	►		
c. Total Print Distribution (Line 15f) + Paid Electronic Copies (Line 16a)	►		
d. Percent Paid (Both Print & Electronic Copies) (16b divided by 16c × 100)	►		

☒ I certify that 50% of all my distributed copies (electronic and print) are paid above a nominal price.

17. Publication of Statement of Ownership

☒ If the publication is a general publication, publication of this statement is required. Will be printed in the NOVEMBER 2021 issue of this publication. ☐ Publication not required.

18. Signature and Title of Editor, Publisher, Business Manager, or Owner

Malathi Samayan - Distribution Controller

Malathi Samayan

Date 9/18/2021

I certify that all information furnished on this form is true and complete. I understand that anyone who furnishes false or misleading information on this form or who omits material or information requested on the form may be subject to criminal sanctions (including fines and imprisonment) and/or civil sanctions (including civil penalties).

PS Form **3526**, July 2014 *(Page 3 of 4)* PRIVACY NOTICE: See our privacy policy on www.usps.com

Moving?

Make sure your subscription moves with you!

To notify us of your new address, find your **Clinics Account Number** (located on your mailing label above your name), and contact customer service at:

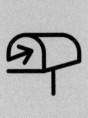

Email: journalscustomerservice-usa@elsevier.com

800-654-2452 (subscribers in the U.S. & Canada)
314-447-8871 (subscribers outside of the U.S. & Canada)

Fax number: 314-447-8029

Elsevier Health Sciences Division
Subscription Customer Service
3251 Riverport Lane
Maryland Heights, MO 63043

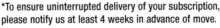

*To ensure uninterrupted delivery of your subscription, please notify us at least 4 weeks in advance of move.

ELSEVIER

Printed and bound by CPI Group (UK) Ltd, Croydon, CR0 4YY

08/05/2025

01864700-0012